THE PSYCHOECOLOGY
OF GLADYS PARLETT

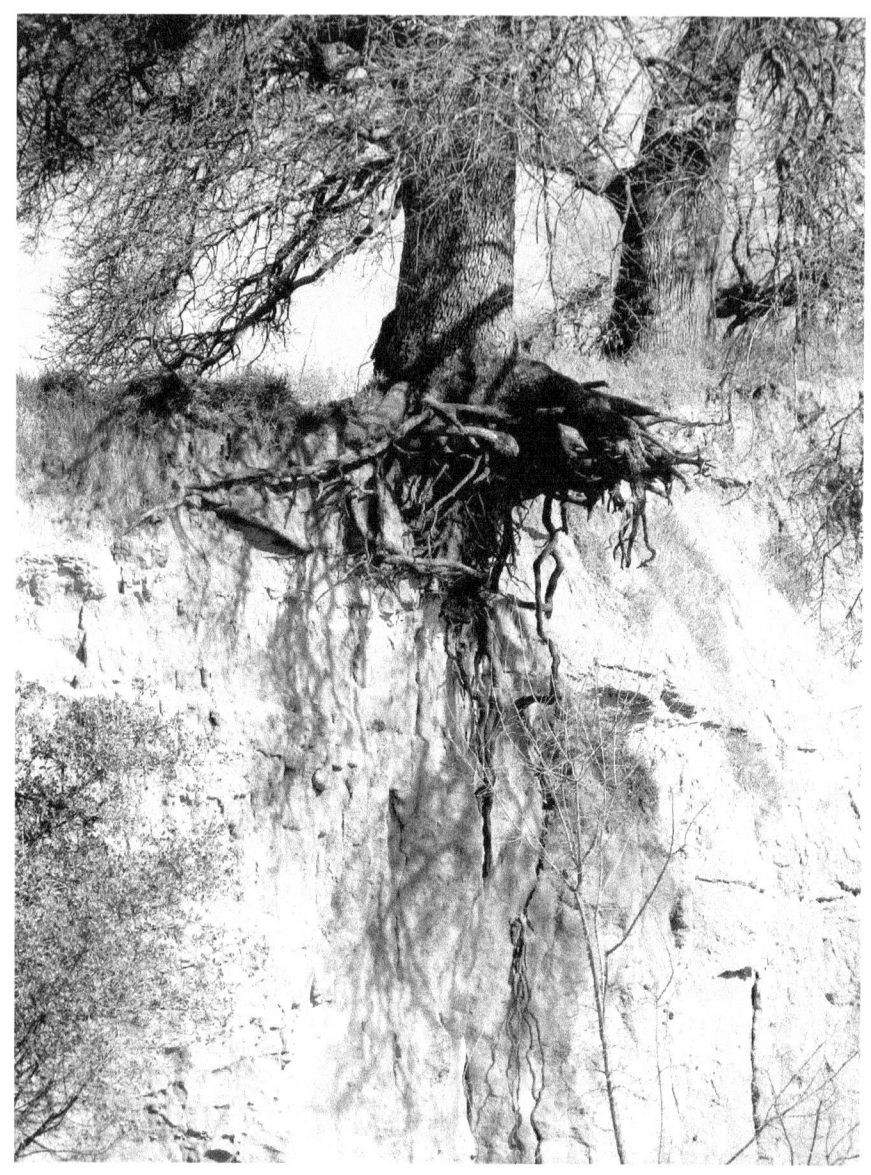

THE PSYCHOECOLOGY OF GLADYS PARLETT

Hidden personal meaning in healthcare

Essays 1976-1990

Volume I:
If you want good personal Healthcare
See a Vet

DAVID ZIGMOND

First published 2015 by New Gnosis Publications
© David Zigmond 2015

The right of David Zigmond to be identified as the author of this
work has been asserted by him in accordance with the Copyright,
Design and Patent Act, 1988

ISBN-13: 978-1515016175
ISBN-10: 151501617X

Printed by CreateSpace

Contents

Introduction

This is a selection of some of my earliest published articles, from 1976-90: a single exception is the dramatically placed heralding first piece, from 2013. It is the first of three volumes. The three make up a triptych. Each though can be readily read separately. All three are also published together, with additional introductory and historical comment, as a large combined volume *If You Want good Personal Healthcare - See a Vet.*

This first volume develops ideas about personal meaning, and how these may be applied throughout healthcare. Since my initial medical training in the 1960s, my interest has evolved into understandings of the more personal and less measurable aspects of my work: how we encounter and make sense of, and to, one another. I have long believed that this kind of understanding, though difficult, is crucial, to our best care. The difficulty is the territory: it is subtle, complex and often elusive – hence the misreading, expedient neglect and oblivion … and then compensating overmanagement: all have become common. The later volumes portray how we are now losing and abandoning this kind of personal understanding, and what the many costs are.

The writing style of these earlier pieces has a formality that deferred to the professional journals of that time. Likewise, some of the details and examples have dated, though these may now add to their interest. What have *not* dated are the motivating and elemental questions and concerns: how may we best make sense of, then positively interact with, one another's wounds, struggles, vulnerability and distress?

The Medical Model of biotechnology has been dramatically and inimitably successful in liberating many areas of our lives previously compromised by pain and loss, fear and haunting. But this success has led us to many secondary problems. For such dazzling potency can also blind: we now often cannot discern the limited range and scope of the objectifying and the biomechanical. Our bedazzlement segues to misuse. This writing explores the confused, troubled yet fertile further reaches beyond those limits.

The articles are generally arranged chronologically, but with one obvious and major exception. I start with a very recent article (*All is Therapy, All is Diagnosis*, 2013) to be followed by the first of the old (*The Medical Model: its limitations and alternatives*, 1976). I have done this to indicate where the earliest ideas may lead, and hoping that the reader may be stimulated to pursue my detailed account of how that happens: the later volumes of this anthology.

Author's note

The oldest writings in this first section date from the 1970s. They comprise a selection of articles written for conventional medical journals. This is reflected in the formal style and some of the medical language and terminology. Amidst this I hope that my early development of humanistic themes – of the experiential, the interpersonal and Holism – will be clear and engaging for the non-medical and current reader.

Readers interested in how specific technical developments have changed patterns and problems of practice over this period will find clear examples. For example, in the last thirty years advances in medication have rendered perforated Peptic Ulcers extremely rare and Auto-immune Arthropathies much more treatable; surgical approaches have transformed the relief and prognosis of Angina. So my examples have dated, but original arguments have not. On balance I decided not to make major revisions, and instead confined rewriting to minor tidying and tightening of some of the text, leaving the form, arguments and examples as they were. If the reader is prepared to accommodate this compromise, current cogency may be combined with historical interest.

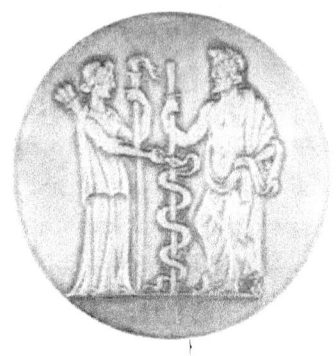

All is Therapy
All is Diagnosis

Unmapped and perishing latitudes of healthcare

.

Advances in medical science have steadily made biomechanical diagnoses and treatments more precise and effective. But this has been achieved, often, by a narrowing of focus so that much human context and meaning becomes unperceived and unconceived. Authentic vignettes from the author's experience – over several decades – illustrate the process and consequences.

'You don't really understand human nature unless you know why a child on a merry-go-round will wave at its parents every time around – and why the parents will always wave back.'
Bill Tammeus, American Journalist (1945-)

1950s. Richness in austerity

The austerity Britain of my childhood sighed wearily: a murky, exhausted wake from the long convulsions of World War II. My surrounding childhood world drew breath amidst a wary stability and peace: many grieved and more were haunted. Less obvious were the wordlessly yet powerfully disturbed: the guilt of the survivors, the partially-sighted resentments of those who sensed infidelities in their absence. My parents – resourceful and uncomplaining people – had their more particular trials and sorrows: my father for a late-war injury which crippled his mobility (and possibly his male self-esteem) for his remaining decades; my mother, much earlier, from her mortally-shattered family who all perished (from 'natural' causes) in her childhood, exposing her as an orphan to the perils of a Depression-ravaged inter-War Britain.

Doctors Paul and Margaret, I think, rapidly sensed and apprised such things even before they knew much of the detail. I remember, as a small boy, feeling protected by their discrete warmth, knowledge and kindness.

Doctors Paul and Margaret were a married couple, our near-neighbours, and together ran a small General Practice from their home. Margaret's consulting room was next to the reception and waiting area. To see Paul we took a few steps outside to a converted garage, where he sat at a handsomely plain and robust oak desk – utility furniture that had served in their thousands throughout the War. The house's domestic hinterland became familiar to me, too: my parents became friendly with Paul and Margaret, I became part of a street-gaggle with their sons.

This interweaving of professional-vocational-locality-domestic-family was, I think, typical of much life – and General Practice – of the time. Amongst better practitioners it led to an unselfconscious integration, an innominate holism, well before common attempts were made to distil, commodify or brand such notions. I think now that Paul and Margaret had a natural understanding – a sense and sensibility – of the unspoken spectres and meanings behind the presented distress or anxiety. Amidst my mists of memory I cannot define clearly the exact times or childhood decisions that led to my later vocations. Yet I think these early experiences, of this couple's benign aura, had a strong inductive influence: even then my innocently receptive eye and mind somehow discerned what I could formulate only much later: that their converged knowledge of the personal and the impersonal could contain, comfort and heal. My early proclivity to such understanding was born of intuition: the vocabulary of scholarship, to describe or explain, would take many more years.

2010s. A small Practice: a bridged island

'The All is alive'

Thales of Miletus (624-527 BC)

Pam knocks gently, knowing my signs of incipient late afternoon gruff fatigue. Her entrance is welcome: she comes revitalising me with hot tea. Pam has been afternoon receptionist in our small practice for a decade. Her middle age experience and deportment are sparkled by youthful gleams and warmly ironic humour. I greet and test her with a long moan of mock-theatrical self-pity conveying the suffering I so self-effacingly endure for others: I, a broken, groaning dying soldier on the carnaged Crimean battlefield; she, the consoling, saintly Florence Nightingale, The Lady with the Tea. Pam's smile is complex: amusement, commiseration, contrition, teasing tolerance and palliation. I do not need to say much: she understands my need for bantered, boundaried, fleeting tenderness. She heals me a little: it has been a long and difficult day. Her tea and resonance may be almost wordless, but they are powerful: like a life-affirming force-field these help contain and sustain me. Such is well-fared welfare; a benign relay – now I am restored to do the same for others.

Pam waits a few seconds for the first signs of my revival, then refreshed attention. Her expression has solemned and now conveys earnest request.

'What now?!' I ask, part question, part peremptory and pre-emptive retort. 'I thought you'd come just to refuel me … It's been a really difficult day.' I add, now more sharply, to scotch any further demands.

'It's Ruby…' Pam persists: she is kind to me, but resilient too. 'I think you should see her today … I've said you will and asked her to wait: she initially didn't want to, but now she will…'

My exasperation is tinged with hostility; I sigh conspicuously: 'But why today, of all days?!' more a warning than a question.

Pam is unerringly calm: 'Because she looks terrible … she's never been right since Robert (her husband) died so quickly of that cancer, just after Christmas … she's always been quiet and shy, but now she's really gone into herself … She comes regularly, every month, for her usual prescriptions. Before she'd chat a little, but now she hardly looks at us … and today I was quite shocked: she's not just withdrawn – she looks really ill: pale and frail … She's all on her own and hates asking for help … Yes, I think you should see her today, while she's here…'

In this small practice people's faces, voices and stories are seen, remembered and recognised. Receptionists accrue percipient and vernacular understandings of patients and their lives. So when longer and good bonds evolve, so do dialogues rich in personal investment.

While doctors' interchanges often segue rapidly to the technical, the task-focused and the managerial, the receptionist's encounters may linger more freely and naturally.

*

Pam is right.

She ushers Ruby in with patient and tender vigilance. Ruby is weak, pale, sallow and almost extinguished of life-spirit. She crosses the room as if impeded by a dense and invisible gas. Despite this torpor she manages her usual self-abnegation – now it is almost inaudible: 'I did ask Pam not to bother you, doctor … I know you've got a lot to do…' Her voice is enfeebled and leaden, her gaze unfocused, dull and lifeless. She is short of breath.

Soon after I am technically categorising and recording. 'Severe Reactive Depression/Impacted Grief. Probably Anaemia ?GI bleeding ?Self-neglect and diet ?Other. Mild Heart Failure.' The medical train is on its tracks. It might not have been if Pam had not looked and thought and cared as she does. Much does not conveniently present as we wish: I must value and protect my receptionists as my social antennae.

I am wondering, too, how could Pam have made this bond of affectionate observation in a now commoner and much larger practice, with its airport-like forms of human processing and (dis)connection? There, I might get home sooner; but what would happen to Ruby?

2010s. A larger Practice: impoverishment in plenty

'Seek knowledge, even if it be in China'

Muhammad

Soon after the new Millennium I sensed my mortality more sharply. I submitted to conventional sense and decided to register with a GP. I, too, will eventually need more than easy (self) prescription for transient complaints: age begins to perish our seals of denial.

I sought and found a small single-handed Practice with a trail of good repute. Dr F. was a likeable, courteous, thoughtful Frenchman; laconic humour spiced an understated compassion. I did not see him much, but each time I did I sensed a growth of joint interest, memory and understanding. Five years ago I was sorrowed by what he told me: he was leaving his work in the NHS and his life in the UK. He had become increasingly frustrated and demoralised by the progressive loss of personal satisfactions, meaning and connections in his work.

He was emigrating to mainland China, to work as a Family Doctor, to reclaim an ethos, a modus vivendum, he increasingly missed. I think my expression signalled perplexity or incredulity, for he rapidly offered bridging explanations: his wife is Chinese, he had spent years learning the language.

I had not needed him much but had sensed a deep affinity, were I to need him. I felt a gentle pang of sadness; I was grieving for a receding attachment I had never really tested, but which I felt had been quietly there.

We shared a warmly farewelling handshake. I briefly thanked him for his friendly and competent contacts with me; I would be sad not to see him again. His look shared this light, sweet flutter of melancholy and he nodded to signal his confluence: 'Of course, there are many people I shall miss, but I think you understand why I am leaving…'

I did and I do.

*

In more recent times my awareness of my blessings has become both stouter and more tremulous: my gratitude for my particular good health is reluctantly laced with a darkening sorrow: for our universal transience – our eventual and inevitable fragility and extinction. I try to be pragmatic; I can offset this a little. I will submit to the nationally vaunted programmes to monitor and control physical risk-factors: horizoned Black Riders of mortality.

*

I attend this re-staffed and managed health centre. A young desultorily expressioned receptionist is looking fixedly at a display on a computer screen. I softly cough to signal my presence, but she is a receptionist who is not receptive. Aware of my waiting presence she attempts to rapidly offload me: 'Over there. Check-in is with the computer', she jerks her head to indicate its direction, keeping unbroken contact with her own computer task.

The computer interrogates and briefs me with brief staccato instructions. When satisfied with my identity and appointment it emits a soft chiming sound to tell me that I am temporarily dismissed and where to go while awaiting further instructions.

I sit in a waiting area that has rows of stackable plastic chairs all facing a wall in which there is a large viewing hatch beyond which the (non) reception staff sit. Above the hatch is a horizontally long, thin, electronic screen across which an endless procession of bannered messages loop to inform, mollify, instruct or warn: 'Feeling down? Find out about our Counselling Services ... Problems with alcohol consumption? ... Are you at risk of HIV? Other sexually transmitted disease? ... Has your child had its MMR vaccinations? ... Stopping smoking will be the one decision you'll never regret ... One consultation is for one patient with one problem ...None of our staff will tolerate any form of rudeness, threat or aggression of any kind. Offending patients are immediately removed from our list ...'. I am aware of the insidious, silent hegemony of such devices; legal civilian nerve-gases to secure compliance and docility.

*

There is a louder, sharper chime, to alert attention. Eyes are raised to the screen to be briefed and instructed. My name appears alongside which consulting room I should go to.

I am seeing the Practice Nurse for some routine blood tests. I have never seen her before. She is looking at a computer as I enter the room, I think to brief her about my 'personal' data. 'Good morning', I say, cheerily, I think. She makes a brief, low, rear-throat sound in acknowledgement. This is wordless and her attention remains with her screen. 'I don't have a request form, but I have come for blood tests: Renal-function, Lipid Profile, Uric Acid and HbAIC'. I say this overtly to inform, but I also have my curiosity about her curiosity, or lack of it: will she enquire about my likely knowledge of such things, and the source of it? She does not.

Instead, without looking, she hurls a question across the room. The question is imperative, stark and unredefinable. The voice is loud, rhetorical and with the guttural, gravelly menace that only impatiently direct Ulster citizens can convey to otherwise benign utterances. 'WHICH ARM?' is the sudden and unframed question. My unprepared, then panicked perception back-somersaults to somewhere in the late-1970s' Northern Ireland: I think I am going to be taken out and shot.

I wince briefly, offer my exposed left arm and then regain sufficient composure to have bland but cordial contact with Nurse Q. As my blood flows I become quietly amused by my images: historical memory-shards, relics of harboured hatreds. Now rapidly recovered I ask whether she is from Northern Ireland. Yes, she says, she was brought up and trained in Londonderry, but her secondary home and family have been here, in London, for many years.

She does not ask me about my probable medical knowledge, or anything else about me. She smiles, as if into a mist, when I leave.

*

I phone the surgery to make an appointment to see the new (for me) GP to discuss my blood tests. I am put on hold while waiting to speak to a receptionist. This administrative hiatus is filled by an expedient plug by and for the practice: a softly, even seductively, authoritative female robotic voice begins to inform me of extra clinics and services that may be offered by the practice, which services can be competently dealt with by nursing staff, and what to do about Out of Hours requirements. In these two minutes I have not yet heard threats or ultimata to the deviants or misbehaved: I am relieved. Another voice cuts in: the real voice of a live receptionist. I make my requests clear, succinct and practical and follow these with some questions about the new order: she replies in kind. 'Dr NP (the new Principal) has expanded the practice and is very busy, so it's easier for you to see one of the part-time assistants. I'll book you to see Dr A: she's very nice…'

*

I come to see Dr A. I do not now expect anyone to recognise or greet me in the practice beforehand. The computer and I, now better acquainted, perform our brief chimed procedure and I go to the waiting area to discern my name from the bannered attempts to crop-spray my mind and conduct.

A more commanding chime now beckons my encounter with Dr A. As I enter she turns a brief, warm but tiredly unfocused smile toward me with a simultaneous 'Hello'. She signals to a chair at the corner of her flimsily veneered, already chipped, new desk before turning away again, back to the computer: the anchor-post for her consultation-consciousness. As she is scrolling down my laboratory results, I can see my non-medical details which remain constant at the top of the changing screen contents. My name is preceded by 'Doctor'.

She turns back to me and offers another jading smile. She asks me how I am: I sense this is mostly a courtesy, but also to ensure I do not have another major agenda before she can start on the one she has decided. I do not have one, so now she is free to quickly move us both onto the problem she has identified and dissected.

'Well, I've looked at your recent blood tests … they're all fine except your sugar, so that's one we have to talk about, because officially you're now a diabetic…'

She goes on to automatically convey structured questions, information and advice about my diet, lifestyle, monitoring regimes and possible future medications. This, I can see, is a generic didactic package she applies to all mild diabetic-risk patients. She has been professionally mannered and clear in her delivery: but it is a delivery and not a dialogue. Fascinatingly (for me) she has learned nothing about me as a person: what kind of life and relationships I have had, what I hope for, what I fear, what brings me joy, what brings me dread – what is likely to sicken me, what to heal me.

Yet within her frame she is a competent didactic teacher, her messages are well rehearsed and well formed. She pauses to see if I understand: I do. I am thoroughly cognisant of what she is telling me: imaginative observation would quickly indicate this. At the end of this auto-piloted freight run she slows a little to tie up this parcel with a faintly simpered, liberal, school-mistress voice: 'Well, I think that's as much as we need to say today – quite a lot, isn't it? – is that ok?' This is a statement and prescription from her, not really a question for me. She tilts her head a little while beaming an unknowing yet coquettish smile: her sweetening and concealment of control is the outer packaging.

She never asks about me being a doctor, and I (partly now for experimental reasons) do not tell her. She shows no curiosity about my personal or occupational life. Dr A acts a role of the agreeably impersonal: I think that she does not know that she does not know me – and can then proceed with her job as if this is of no consequence to either of us.

At present this is, arguably, enough: I do not yet have the kind of dis-ease, disease, dependence or infirmity which requires the kind of personal understandings that can contain, comfort and heal. If I live long enough, I will.

Yes, Dr A's advice is sound, and her prescribed medications far more precise and powerful than anything that was available to my 1950s doctors. Yes, *treatment* is usually much better, but what about *care*? Here there is no such commensurate progress, often the reverse. I know that when my health and life begin to ineluctably unravel, like Ruby, I will want *personal* and personal-*continuity* of care from practitioners with that ethos and vocation: people like Doctors Paul and Margaret.

But in a healthcare world increasingly designed, commissioned, commodified, commercialised and managed by others very different from them, and remote from me, how is this possible? What, instead, will happen?

The portents are already visible, if only we will look.

*

Healthcare is a humanity guided by science.

Ω

'The danger of the past was that men became slaves. The danger of the future is that men become robots.'

Erich Fromm, *The Sane Society*, 1955

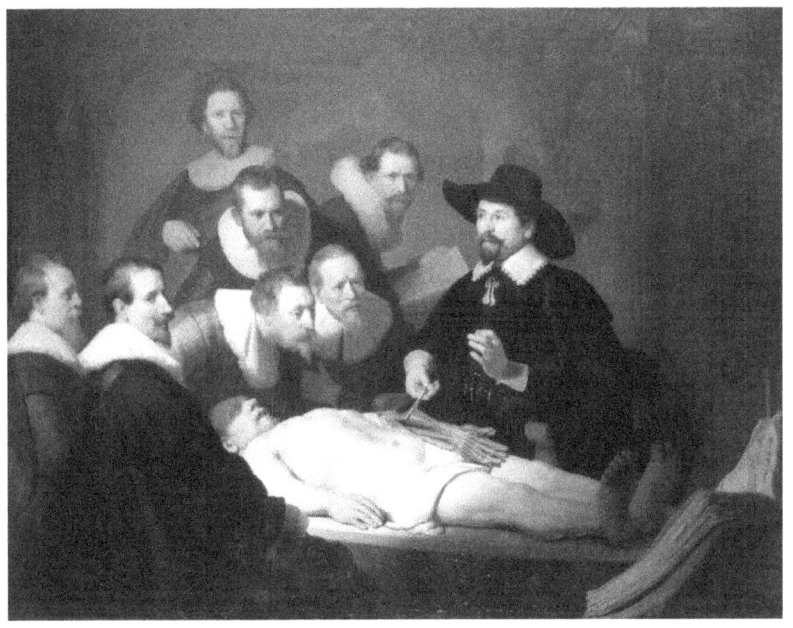

Rembrandt *The Anatomy Lesson of Dr. Nicolaes Tulp* 1632

The Medical Model
– its Limitations and Alternatives

How humanism may synergise biomechanism

What is the Medical Model?

Although most doctors' working time is spent using the Medical Model, we might find the term difficult to define. This itself reflects particular restrictions of thinking: those conditioned by years of training and modelling ourselves on other doctors. We then find it difficult to stand outside our methodological framework and see other realities.

Here is a preliminary definition: the Medical Model assumes a simple mechanical view of illness and the body it occurs in. Any illness is thus seen simply as a fault in the machine. Although lip-service may be paid to interfering concepts of the mind, the family and the environment, these are uncomfortable bedfellows of the Medical Model and the machine-body continues to be regarded as something that functions autonomously: a hermetic system. Diagnoses therefore tend to be formulated in terms of structural or functional failures of the machine alone. It follows that because treatment methods derive from diagnostic concepts, then medical treatment is likely to be equally mechanistic and exclusive of non-material or psychological factors. The Medical Model sometimes does well with these restrictions: for example, in orthopaedic trauma surgery where the problems are most clearly circumscribed and structural.

The Reasons We Use the Medical Model

The Medical Model has enticing clarity: it is generally succinct, tangible and understandable: it has easy confluence with a scientific method which relies primarily on objective and measurable observation. This has the advantage of offering terminology, formulations and explanations which can (seemingly) be unambiguously understood and then handled in an identical fashion by all similarly trained people. We therefore have the potential of knowing precisely what others are talking about and what they are doing in defined situations. This makes possible the kinds of standardisation of terminology and concepts that are essential for scientific communication and research. These activities can then give us useful information about general patterns of illness and the effectiveness of therapies.

Less defensible reasons for our inflexible and often inept use of the Medical Model lie in habit and conditioning. Most of us were never encouraged or taught to use anything else. Therefore we have developed skills only within a narrow framework: this we continue to use alone, even when a problem requires alternative or additional methods.

Some Snares We Fall into Unconsciously

At its best the Medical Model functions extremely well, providing guidelines for processing circumscribed problems and predicting what the outcome will be, with or without intervention. Such important considerations are invoked in the concept of diagnosis. Diagnosis provides powerful navigational aid when we have substantial knowledge about what we are labelling: *Substantial diagnosis*. If, on the other hand, a diagnosis does not offer us accurate information about prognosis and intervention, then we can call this a *Nominal diagnosis* because it gives only an arcane name to something we know very little about. Let us take an example of each.

1. Acute follicular beta-haemolytic streptococcal tonsillitis is a Substantial diagnosis. It tells us with relative certainty what the symptoms and signs are, what treatment is going to be effective and what the hazards are of leaving the complaint untreated. The Medical Model works well here. Our concepts and tools are effective. We know what to do and are rarely surprised by subsequent events if we do the right thing. The patient senses this, and he and the doctor will probably get along well in this situation.

2. Non-articular or seronegative rheumatoid arthritis*[1] is a Nominal diagnosis. It really does not tell us much at all. It does not tell us how the patient's health will be affected in the future. In five years' time he may be perfectly well despite not having any treatment. On the other hand he may be crippled with arthritis, blind with iritis and have an ileostomy because of fulminating ulcerative colitis. Furthermore, he may have developed all this despite the best treatment available. The Medical Model is now working extremely badly. The doctor feels unsure and ineffective and is likely to be on the defensive. The patient senses this and reciprocally lacks confidence. The relationship between patient and doctor is now likely to be more strained. The patient may become 'difficult and demanding'. The doctor attempts to maintain a confident persona by whatever new kinds of investigation and therapy he can think of, because he does not know what else to offer.

Substantial and Nominal Diagnosis

The two diagnoses here are really quite different in their implication. The 'Substantial diagnosis' offers us extremely helpful information as to what we might do and what we should expect, while the 'Nominal diagnosis' does neither satisfactorily. At best it is a descriptive tag which we attach to some apparently similar phenomena which we do not understand. However, such is the power of words that we equate them with understanding. Just as a religious incantation is intended to dispel evil spirits or attract good ones, so the

---

[1] *Post-scripted note December 2014. In the thirty-eight years since this was written, scientific knowledge has advanced, so that these conditions are now more contained with Substantial (rather than Nominal) diagnoses. Thus the knowledge has grown – the examples are now somewhat obsolete – but the guiding principles remain.

Rather than rewrite the examples, they are retained for historical interest. It is hoped that the underlying argument is unobscured. It remains seminal to this book.

medical incantation of naming the diagnosis is meant to dispel uncertainty and indecision. However, as we can see from the above example it often fails to do this – nevertheless we continue to repeat the ritual and hope the rest will follow.

Many ailments fall somewhere between the Substantial and Nominal end of the diagnostic spectrum. Often a particular illness will shift its position at different times. For example, a man who has the dyspepsia appropriate to a barium-meal proven duodenal ulcer* may well present the doctor with a Nominal diagnosis, as the course of his illness and the efficacy of therapy remain largely unknown. If this same man perforates his ulcer then the situation is one where a Substantial diagnosis becomes very important; treatment is incontrovertible and clear-cut and the prognosis with and without this intervention equally so.

In formulating diagnoses we need to be aware of their position on this spectrum. Are we really making meaningful statements, or are we merely tagging labels onto phenomena we are ignorant about? If it is the latter, who is benefited by the Nominal diagnosis – the doctor, the patient or the institution? Complex terminology is often used as a defence against substantial ignorance. If the doctor is lost, bemused and largely ineffective, then at least he can fall back on some technical words and 'scientific' concepts which he hopes will maintain his position in his own and the patient's eyes as the potent and unassailable authority. Such unconscious defences and collusions are not always a bad thing, but they can often block the doctor's opportunities to explore more fruitful avenues of rapport and investigation.

What the Medical Model Misses Out

Because it has its roots in the scientific method, the Medical Model functions best when incorporating phenomena that are measurable and quantifiable. That is, it copes well with the physical or organic components of illness, but has much less assurance with other factors, the most important of which are personal and psychological. Most of us are instinctively aware of the importance of external stresses and inner emotional conflicts in the precipitation, course and eventual outcome of many illnesses. Yet the problem of being unable to directly measure stress or emotional conflict is always problematic.

There have certainly been attempts to rate and scale such reactions as fear (anxiety) and dispiritedness (depression), but on scrutiny these endeavours only measure phenomena which are assumed to have a direct relationship with the inner experience, which itself remains elusive and unmeasurable to our tools of scientific enquiry. True, we can measure and classify certain of the simpler aspects of behaviour – that is, reported speech and habits, alcohol consumption, compulsive rituals etc – but never the inner life that motivates them. Rating scores of described experiences are beset with ambiguities and potential distortions. If the usual Medical Model is incapable of dealing imaginatively with these aspects of illness then we have two alternatives. We can ignore the non-organic, non-measurable aspects of medicine and remain always within the respectable territory of scientific convention, or we can use alternative modes and models – we can add to the more traditional medical diagnoses.

Such a whole-person or even whole-family approach to illness has received increasing attention in recent years. Perhaps the most influential work in this area pertinent to the general practitioner was investigated by Michael Balint. Much of his work indicates that the traditional medical diagnosis used alone is often severely limited in the amount of help it gives to the doctor in understanding the patient's illness, what he can do about it, and what he might expect in the future. Balint found that these limitations can be countered by the doctor entering into new, speculative territory where skills of empathetic imagination might attempt to formulate the position of illness within its matrix of family relationships and internal emotional tensions. Such formulations cannot give us the same sort of uniform agreement of the more traditional diagnoses, but this venture offers much else in terms of understanding and influence. The following case illustrates a typical medical formulation, then expanded by humanistic speculation.

A Case from General Practice

Mr CT is 65 years of age. One month before his date of retirement he developed ankle oedema and ascites. His general practitioner first saw him late one night when he developed acute and severe dyspnoea. Examination indicated mild hypertension, biventricular cardiac failure and slight cardiac enlargement. Routine investigations yielded only the one additional useful finding that his cardiac failure was probably caused by ischaemic heart disease (ECG evidence). Unfortunately, fairly large doses of Digoxin and diuretics had no effect on his ascites and oedema, although his blood pressure was well controlled with Methyldopa. He had no further attacks of pulmonary oedema.

One month later, therefore, he was hospitalised with a view to controlling his right-sided heart failure. Even with complete bed rest and massive doses of Frusemide and Spironolactone this problem was extremely difficult to manage. At this time he became increasingly anxious, irritable and demanding. It became difficult to keep him in bed or to get him to take his medication, which he seemed to view with suspicion. Eventually this ended in a mixed manic-paranoid reaction. He claimed to be in perfect health and said that he was in hospital to help his wife's illness (she was in good health).

While embarking on numerous impractical projects simultaneously, he would make grandiose and untrue proclamations about how wealthy and important he was. His distractibility made it difficult for him to sleep or eat, and his motor restlessness made him a difficult nursing problem. At times he showed fluctuating paranoid delusions about the nursing staff, saying that they had poisoned him and stolen his money. On the other hand he became unprecedentedly sexually suggestive and familiar with the same nurses. Although showing undoubted manic signs when interviewed, the depression was just below the surface. He became extremely distressed and tearful when certain important and personal and life topics were discussed. Although Chlorpromazine was needed to contain the immediate situation, the bulk of his improvement came from helping him come to terms with his underlying emotional problems.

Before we move into this alternative and personal diagnostic area, we might formulate the medical diagnoses thus: mild controlled hypertension with ischaemic heart disease causing decompensated right ventricular failure. Superadded mixed manic-paranoid psychosis.

Method or Madness?

Let us now look into the story of this man's life and see how his illness fits in. The hallmarks of Mr CT's life were caution, safety, orderliness and continence. He only took the minimum and essential risks in life, and then only with the maximum preparation. He had married 40 years ago and had lived in the same house ever since. Throughout these four decades, he had worked in the same clerical job, though with minor promotions. In his work he was diligent to the point of obsession and found any criticism or disorder highly disturbing. His marriage was contained in a similar framework of orderliness and safety. His wife never worked outside the home because he found the idea threatening. Their life together was safely but drably concordant, and structured by well-worn routine. Their sexual life sounded courteously suppressed and obscured: latterly he had been rendered impotent, probably because of his Methyldopa.

His leisure time similarly drifted: passive and unexplorative. He watched television indiscriminately and fell asleep after supper while reading the *Daily Express*. Occasionally he would potter in the garden, but took little else in the way of physical activity. His lack of pursued hobbies or interests led to boredom and irritability at weekends: time and freedom became enemies. Anger was never overt; he would similarly avoid or appease any conflict, which he evidently found threatening. In his social relationships he had cordial but ritualised contacts, hence no committed or intimate friends. Because of his passivity and temerity, he felt exploited at work: a cruel consequence of his diligence and compliance. He was resentful that after 40 years of service to his employers, he left with little promotion, perfunctory compliments and a gold watch. Secretly he had hoped for grand applause and a big send-off.

Last, but not least, this man had never been seriously ill.

Understanding and Management

How does this backcloth help us in our understanding and engagement with this frightened and frustrated man? One of the most striking features about him is his inability to assert himself as an individual, or act in any way that would lead to dissonance with others. His early background can help us understand. He experienced his father as authoritarian, overpowering, distant yet violent when drunk or frustrated. His mother and siblings learned that the only way to be safe was to be silent, obedient and unnoticed. He had carried this legacy of submissive, stoic resentment throughout the rest of his life.

Until the onset of his illness.

In his fantasy life he had vaguely hoped that retirement would bring some of the fulfilment and satisfaction that had always eluded him. The reality turned out to be very different. Even without his illness, his fixation to many years' routine, his inflexibility and lack of creative interests made retirement an extremely demanding testing-ground for this overadapted and underdeveloped man. It is even possible that he recognised this unconsciously, and that his heart-failure represented a lost battleground: the disconsolate 'loss of heart' – that this was all there was to his life.

What is evidently true is that his serious illness then brought to consciousness the possible imminence of his death. This insinuated the futility of his life: all the things he wished he had achieved, yet had avoided. Such a demeaned view of his life was intolerable: a defence was essential. Hence his manic reaction; thence his grandiosity, his multiple and unrealistic plans, his display of hypersexuality and the demanding urges he had kept so well contained for so many years. Equally difficult for him was the way in which physical illness had underlined his shamed self-perception of passivity and weakness; hence the denial that he himself was ill, and that any illness within him was displaced from his wife, or the result of others poisoning him.

Other destabilising facets emerged: the established structure of his marriage had been radically changed. Although a sedentary man, he had claimed the conventionally undisputed dominant marital role: his submissive wife offered him some sense of domestic power. His illness, however, had reversed their roles. Now he was the partner who had to stay at home and be provided for – her role until he fell ill.

He struggled painfully and tearfully with coming to terms with these realities. With a growing sorrowful calm he perceived how his mania and paranoia were defences against his deep-rooted frustrations and sense of loss. It was bravado in the face of grief. He was both grieving and raging for the life he had feared to live, and whose possibilities were now passing.

The human core of this formulation lies outside conventional scientific and medical methods. It can neither be proved nor disproved, because his feelings and his entire inner world cannot be objectively observed or measured. With unprovable plausibility they can be logically inferred; with imagination, intuitively felt. Yet without this meeting in the regions of uncertainty he must endure his grief, fear and primitive anger alone. Enabling him to share these brought compassionate palliation and relief. His manic and paranoid defences became no longer necessary.

Understanding his rage enabled him to metabolise it. He has then been freer to cope with his diminished and disabled life. Although sorrowful he is not now 'ill' in the strict psychiatric sense. Interestingly his heart failure became much better controlled. Has his cardiac function improved because his heart is no longer subject to the autonomic-nervous and hormonal storms that beset it in his previous state of emotional turbulence? Happily he no longer needs major tranquillisers to assure his sanity and stability: his inner healing has now anchored this.

Conclusion

This case illustrates how the Medical Model can be integrated within a wider framework of alternatives. From a strict scientific view these other concepts do not avail themselves so readily to more direct kinds of empirical testing. Yet the price of ignoring these alternatives is high. Mr CT would probably have continued his mania, paranoia and depression and had a much more turbulent end of life. It is likely, too, that his cardiac failure would have remained intractable: his improvement was definite and otherwise unaccountable.

Such pursuits are subtle: they require more flexibility in approach than we are generally trained for. In return our understanding of, and rapport with, the whole patient becomes richer. The benefits extend beyond prevention or curtailment of significant illness in others – we ourselves derive greater human interest and satisfaction from our work.

$$\Omega$$

Published in *Hospital Update* 424-427, Aug.1976

Illness as Strategy
and Communication

In spite of the vast bulk of literature deriving from psychoanalysis and applicable to medicine, the predominant orientation in the training and practice of doctors remains entrenched in concepts of illness which are mechanistic and unconnected with the patient's emotional and relationship matrix. Perhaps the increasing precision and sophistication of our technology has made other dimensions of illness seem less important in assessment and management.

Modern techniques of diagnosis and therapy are now complex, powerful and, at times, dangerous. Because of these developments, it is hardly surprising that the contemporary doctor may see himself as some kind of biological engineer or technician, whose job it is to rectify faults in the human machine. However, there are emotional factors which are also operative in maintaining this kind of technocracy and alienation between patient and doctor. We can think of these as 'defences' whose function is to protect both parties against distressing and threatening feelings, and also conserve the doctor's position of executive power. I have explored some of these factors in an earlier paper (Zigmond 1977) but here I want to elaborate further the role of illness in meeting the emotional needs of patients. Without this approach, I believe, diagnosis and therapy are often liable to be less effective. Four cases are described later to illustrate this.

Illness as Strategy

Illness is usually conceived and experienced as a malevolent intrusion by an alien force, which has no connection with the self and its relationship with others. Whatever our knowledge of the mechanics, the illness is felt and thought of as something apart, that strikes us 'out of the blue'. Because of this split we feel that we are at the mercy of the disease process, which seems to have an autonomous, even magical, existence. In the face of illness, therefore, we are all liable to feel helpless and dependent, either on the disease process or on any person who may alleviate it. In psychoanalytic jargon, disease may be said to be 'ego-dystonic', i.e. separate from the familiar complex of volition and experience that we conceive of as 'the self'. Such infirmity, therefore, may compromise our usual traits of independence and individual effectiveness. When ill, we often find ourselves incapable of making decisions or performing the necessary tasks to realize them. A state of regression is engendered, where autonomy is necessarily abdicated. If a man in his 40s, for example, is admitted to a coronary care unit, it is likely that he will be necessarily regressed to the early infant stage. He will be put to bed, washed, and evacuate himself into a bottle or bedpan. Such dramatic and coerced regression may be difficult, but any resistance on his part is likely to have him branded as 'uncooperative'.

Alternatively, however, illness may have its uses. There is a childlike and dependent part in us all, whatever our age or maturity. From the infants we all were, there remains our archaic and relentless drive for recognition, attention and care from those around us. Equally, we may at times feel immense rage and destructiveness towards those who are closest, just as the infant does rather more overtly. Because of societal taboos, such intense dependence or rage is clearly discouraged. Illness, however, is a state where the individual is not thought to be responsible for himself, and thus offers a less stigmatizing and more conventionally acceptable means of regressing into this child-system. Under the cloak of illness we may become helpless, ask others to look after us, act out and abdicate our usual identity-structure. Behaviour which in other circumstances would be criticized or even punished, can be connived at, and often colluded with.

Illness as Communication

It has already been indicated in which way illness may serve as a conventionally acceptable route to regression that might otherwise be considered dys-social or antisocial. This does not mean, however, that illness communicates only archaic and primitive messages. Very commonly an individual has developed his own specific taboos with particular kinds of feelings. Frequently this is because his parents indicated to him that these feelings would be ignored, belittled or even punished. Such moulding of emotional responses occurs via parental influence in a child's formative years. Explicit pressures such as punishment or mockery are clear, but covert pressures such as a hostile tone of voice or parental indifference are commoner, though sometimes equally damaging. The feelings that are forbidden may range from fear to assertion, from sadness to anger, depending on the parents' area of difficulty. Later on in life this person will be unable to express this particular feeling with direct words and gestures. Instead he will resort to oblique expressions via somatic language which, in his developmental frame of reference, provides immunity from the hurt he received when he was young. In this way psychosomatic illness may be viewed as having its roots in a habitual and compulsive form of body language.

Case No. 1: A Little Boy Escapes Bellyaching

Stephen, aged seven, is generally a healthy boy who has a good communication with his humorous and intelligent mother. His parents separated when he was an infant. Mother has recently remarried. Stephen is tentatively fond of her new husband but feels insecure with him. In addition, Stephen's real father has fallen into debt and depression and has been unable to pay the usual maintenance, creating an atmosphere of tension and split loyalties for Stephen, who is fond of his father, and has regular contact with him. Because of father's difficulties, he had to defer his weekend visit. The following dialogue then ensued.

Stephen: (plaintively) 'Mum, I feel sick and I've got a tummy ache.'

Mother: (intuitively, noting his empty dinner plate) 'I am sorry Stephen, it's horrible isn't it? . . . I think you're sad and disappointed that daddy's not happy and he can't come today. But it doesn't mean he doesn't love you... I think your tummy ache is saying that you're a bit angry and sad.' Stephen then goes to his mother, sits on her lap, has a cuddle and forgets his abdominal discomfort.

Mother here did not discount Stephen's tummy ache, but more importantly she recognized, validated and accepted his sadness, anger and confusion. Contrast this with a possible and likely alternative:

Stephen: 'Mum, I feel sick and I've got a tummy ache.'

Mother: 'Oh dear, I do hope it's nothing bad . . . you must go to bed, and I'll call the doctor straight away.'

Here the long-term and short-term outcomes are likely to be quite different. Mother only takes Stephen's stomach ache seriously because she herself cannot cope with unhappy and distressed feelings. Her implicit message to Stephen is, 'I don't mind you having stomach ache, but don't show me your unhappiness, because I don't know how to deal with it'. Stephen now learns that overt communication of distress, anger and sadness cannot be displayed; he must settle for tummy ache instead, if he is to evoke mother's protection and concern. As an adult he may well be getting antacids from his general practitioner every time his dyspepsia indicates sadness and frustration that he feels inwardly compelled to bear alone. In this latter situation, the alert and empathetic general practitioner will be able to verbalize and accept the patient's distress and frustrations, thereby rendering them more tolerable to the patient himself. The doctor who is able to recognize, validate and hold a patient's unhappiness, performs much the same function as a parent with a child who is afraid of being overwhelmed by the intensity of his feelings. Once confirmed and shared, some resolution or subsidence of emotional problems may be possible. This is a cornerstone of psychotherapy at every level of practice.

Case No. 2: Illness as Rebellion in an Over-ordered Family

Miss VH is 23 years of age. Since the age of 16 she has suffered from well-documented episodes of mania. All but her last hospitalization were to an organically orientated psychiatric unit, where a wide span of major tranquillizers and Lithium was tried, which may have quelled the acute crises, but seemed to have little prophylactic effect on her disability.

Her last admission was to a less organically orientated unit, but followed the same cacophonous pattern. On arrival she showed clinical signs of mania in her psychomotor acceleration, distractibility, emotional liability, prickliness, grandiose and discursive thinking, and so forth. However, the doctor sensed her underlying sadness and despair. He offered her his observation saying, 'It seems to me that underneath all this you're feeling really miserable and helpless'. She stayed silent for some time and her mania seemed to evaporate giving way to a rather sad and confused child. 'Yes', she replied, 'nobody ever listens to me at home, especially my father, so I get angry and they say, "Oh, she's getting ill again, we'd better call the doctor". And he's always on their side. He doesn't listen either, so I have to come into hospital again.' By inference it seemed that VH came from a household where anger and rebellion could not be expressed directly, only through illness – in this case mania. It emerged that VH is an only child, from a stable, professional and rather joyless marriage. Her father is a rigid, authoritarian, ex-military man whose need for order and obedience seemed indefatigable. Mother has learned to adapt through subdued compliance and stamina, but VH never managed this so successfully. Father's moralism and strictures with VH's social life indicated difficulties with his own sexual feelings, and possibly some incestuous impulses towards VH

It was only through acknowledging her very real anger, and frustration with her coerced dependence, that she was able to organize her emotional resources to deal with the problem realistically. In spite of her fear and pain she has now left home, is off her drugs and is forging her own identity slowly but surely. These substantial gains were demanding and difficult: she made good use of skilled professional guidance. Her manic 'illness' symbolized her battle for autonomy and has not returned.

Case No. 3: A Desperate Struggle for Recognition in Infancy

Baby Kevin F. was aged five months on admission. His birth and first three months had been physically uneventful. For two months, however, he had been restless and posseted all his feeds, so that he had lost weight dramatically. On admission he was evidently very ill; his weight was on the third percentile, he was extremely frail and dehydrated, as attested by his sunken fontanelle, dry tongue and raised blood urea. His history was against congenital pyloric stenosis, and barium studies failed to show a hiatus hernia. In physical terms his diagnosis was one of rumination syndrome – he had no physical lesion, but was bringing back his food for self-gratification and to evoke contact with others.

The family and emotional diagnosis was more difficult and complex. His parents were an intelligent and ambitious couple, and this was their first child. Mother was an insecure and prickly woman, who escaped the conflictual relationship with her short-tempered father by getting married to a man who was very much like him. Mr and Mrs F. thus lived in a state of competitive discord, and Mrs F. harbours extensive grievances against men because she feels they will control her and usurp her independence. She had been doing well in her career as a teacher, and became pregnant ambivalently with pressure from her husband. Because of her feelings about the men in her life, she secretly hoped for a baby girl with whom she could develop an alliance of women.

With the birth of Kevin she felt bitterly disappointed, and found herself unable to give him the maternal and nurturing responses that were necessary. Kevin was fed, bathed and bedded efficiently, but was never played with or enjoyed. He would sit in this pristine cot wanting to explore or be loved, but mother sat silently and sullenly doing *The Times* crossword puzzle. Kevin's progress in hospital was dramatic. He was played with, chatted to and smiled at by the nurses, and his feeding difficulties soon settled, with the attendant improvement in weight. Mrs F. recognized her lack of nurturing, where it came from, and how it led to Kevin's severe illness. Fortunately, Mr and Mrs F. were able to embark on, and co-operate with, a mixture of individual and marital therapy, which brought about a greater fulfilment in their marriage, and a disappearance of Kevin's desperate strategies to be loved and related to.

Case No. 4: Illness as an Escape Mechanism

Mr G. K. is aged 53 years. He had been physically healthy all his life until a number of apparently physical crises were brought to the attention of his general practitioner, and then the medical and casualty departments of the local hospital. Over several months he had a number of alarming attacks, consisting of tightness in the chest, a feeling of impending suffocation, paraesthesiae in the arms and hands and prostrating weakness and dizziness. Suspected cardiac and respiratory disease was never confirmed, but he continued to be subject to these crises, with the consequent hospitalizations and investigations. The only positive physical finding was a persistent mild idiopathic hypertension (BP 170/110). Eventually the recognition of these episodes as panic attacks led to an exploration of his underlying problems.

Mr G. K. is a Greek Cypriot but has spent most of his adult life in this country, has married an English woman and now has three teenage children. Early on in his life Mr G. K. decided that he must be strong, ignore his own feelings but look after other people, whom he needed to perceive as less strong than himself. He learned this life-role as a child because of his parents' own marital difficulties. Father was a large and unhappy man whose resentment with his lot was largely projected onto his wife and children via displays and acts of violence. These were exacerbated by his drinking and gambling, which gave mother an excuse to persecute him, thereby perpetuating the vicious circle. Although he might physically assault mother, he would stop short of this with his children. Mr G. K. learned, as a small boy, that he could rescue his mother by interposing himself between his parents. However, to do this he had to be able to deny his own fear of the situation. As a child of six years he learned that his mother's survival depended on his rescuing her with his bravado and fearlessness. This role was pursued relentlessly despite the circumstantial changes in his life. Father died and he came to England with his mother, where he soon met his future wife. Although his new family was under no real duress, he still felt the compulsion to be the never-failing rescuer and provider. He was a warm and caring man, but could only show this by working 'for the family' to the extremes of his physical endurance, and by taking on a firm patriarchal role in the belief that his family could never function autonomously without him. This hero at war was not an easy man to love at home; he and his wife insidiously became emotionally and sexually estranged.

It was the Turkish invasion of Cyprus that brought forward the collapse of this man's outdated and cumbersome defences. His home town was destroyed, and with it many friends and relatives who together formed so much of his emotional roots. His grief and hurt were enormous, but because of his lifelong bravado and denial of weakness or feeling he was unable to acknowledge these to himself, even less be comforted by others. In an effort to escape his feelings of impotence and loss, he worked at the expense of even more time and energy. Eventually this defence also became inadequate and led to his panic attacks. Although his taboo on verbal communication of distress made this initially impossible, the message in his panic attacks was quite clear. His pent-up feelings of loss, despair, fear and powerlessness were all evident in his cries, his choking and trembling. Here was powerful somatic communication, while his tongue had not yet permission to speak. Psychotherapy with this man has been brief and gratifying. Encouraging him to acknowledge, re-own and share his vulnerabilities and feelings has abolished his unwitting strategy of illness, and brought about much emotional growth in his family and marital life.

Medically it is noteworthy that he has reverted to being normotensive, and is now maintaining this without his hypotensive drugs. Such exploration and therapy of his somatic communications has hopefully freed him of the need to be ill in order to express and work through his distress. The absence of such intervention could have resulted in a much more real and physically damaging cardiovascular catastrophe.

Conclusion

We are all an amalgam of what we consider to be creditable and discreditable qualities – what we wish to be, and what we fear we may be. Generally we are conditioned to thinking that 'good' qualities are those such as strength, autonomy, generosity and courage. However, there is a child-system of percepts and feelings in everyone which confronts us with our intense and primitive feelings of rage, destructiveness, infantile passivity and the wish to be taken care of. This infant part of ourselves remains active, but discouraged from expression by societal taboos. Some families, also, have more particular taboos with other feelings, such as fear and sadness. Because all these feelings are powerful but not allowed direct expression, they must be split off and expressed, covertly, leaving the rest of the apparent personality intact. Illnesses of many kinds offer such a system of strategy and communication; this not only applies to psychiatric and hysterical syndromes, but also to very tangible organic reactions such as duodenal ulceration and asthma. Although alternative skills are required to understand the language of illness, the results are often gratifying, and at times may even be lifesaving.

$$\Omega$$

Reference
Zigmond, D. *Update,* 1977, 15, 159.

Bibliographical Note
Nothing said about the relationship aspects of medicine would be complete without reference to the contribution of Michael Balint. His book *The Doctor, his Patient and the Illness* (Pitman Medical 1968) is now an established classic. I have also found the concepts of Transactional Analysis invaluable in formulating the developmental and transactional basis of illness as a form of communication. The following books provide an excellent introduction to this system of psychology:

Berne, E, *Games People Play,* Penguin, Harmondsworth, Middx, 1967
Berne, E. *What do You Say After You Say Hello?,* Corgi Books, London, 1975
Harris, T. *I'm OK – You're OK,* Pan, London, 1973
Steiner, C. *Scripts People Live,* Grove Press, London, 1974

Published in *Update* 1977

Adjustment or Change?

Radical Issues in Psychiatry

Author's post-scripted foreword (March 2014)

'Adjustment or change?' was written in 1977 and is republished here, nearly four decades later, in its original form.

It is writing very much of its period: political debate was more sanguine and polarised, old fashioned socialism looked set for longevity (and the USSR for eternity). Vietnam was a fresh, sharp memory. Feminism was young, raw and accelerating. There was more righteous anger, optimism and political diversity.

Although this period-piece may now, in places, sound callow and strident, it still has important messages. Although theorists, politicians and planners are often now very mindful of the importance of social and environmental factors in the generation of illness, this is often not evident on the hospital ward-round, or in the doctor's consulting room. The contemporary practitioner is likely to confine his view to looking into two 'boxes': the patient (the locus of biomechanical breakdown) and the computer (for the abstracted data). Doctors now are likely to be less personally acquainted with a particular patient, their story, their social milieu and their physical environment. Doctor-patient interactions are now likely to be even more myopically confined to the biomechanical, and devoid of the kind of personal influences that create a broader view of growth and healing.

This article, for all its gauche rhetoric, is probably more relevant now than in 1977. Equally arresting are these considerations: where in the NHS could Mrs E (Patient 2) get such undesignated therapy?, and: what mainstream medical journal would now risk publishing such feral dissent from the frontline?

I can well remember my surprise and confusion when, as a medical student, I discovered the irrelevance of medical technology in the epidemiological patterns of tuberculosis. Until that time I had assumed that technical advances in diagnosis and management had been central to its decline. Like many aspiring professionals, I had imagined and wished my power to be far greater than it was.

The medical model and social perspectives

To find that the overwhelming bulk of tuberculosis was more dependent on our arrangements for living together than on mass radiography, Mantoux testing or streptomycin, brought me acute awareness of how distorting the hospital and individual centred models of medicine can be. I learned far more about diagnosis and management of individual pathology than about the social framework that led to overcrowding, cold, damp and malnutrition. Poverty was parcelled, with an apology of scientific correctness, into 'social classes V and VI'. True, I was training to be a doctor, not a political radical, but I wonder how many doctors continue to be similarly oblivious, or indifferent, to the fundamental social forces operative in patterns of 'illness'.

Illness as a scapegoat

The concept of illness may very often be seen as a way of 'scapegoating' a part of a problem so that the presenting patient is labelled, treated and despatched, leaving the forces acting on him unexamined or unchallenged. Tuberculosis sanatoria may have contained some individual cases of consumption, but were no substitute for proper working or living conditions. In this respect, treating the designated patient alone, while ignoring the pathogenic influences acting on him, can be seen as a kind of sop, or parrying manoeuvre. It is similar to the unhappy or ill family, whose discord is clearly related to alienating and depressing housing, who are told: "The council can't find you a decent home, but they'll send a social worker to see you instead". The social worker's implicit brief here is to act as a decoy and tranquillizer, so that the immediate symptoms of disturbance can be averted, if not suppressed. Perhaps she will have the skill to transmute a housing problem into 'casework' or 'family therapy'; the important point is, however, that she cannot provide a new house, only social work skills.

In formulating and dealing with symptomatology within the conceptual framework of individual pathology, it is easy to make the assumption that the only fault lies within the patient, not in the world in which he lives. Studies in social medicine and statistics may provide a theoretical antidote to such projection, but the actual practice of medicine and other caring agencies continues to enact this conservative principle. So long as we describe certain people as being 'ill', rather than oppressed or injured, the rest of us can feel blameless and unquestioning of the status quo.

Illness and psychiatry

Nowhere is this concept more relevant but concealed than in psychiatry. At the present time this is exhibited most floridly and distastefully in the USSR, but the West has its insidious counterpart, which is probably equally extensive. Such a view has been elaborated from different aspects by Reich, Szasz, Laing and Illich. For the general practitioner, the extrapolation of variety and quantity of psychotropic drug consumption, while 'psychiatric morbidity' continues to rise is perhaps a more vivid and understandable illustration of these principles. In my earliest experiences of general practice I felt like the bewildered King Canute, trying to turn back waves of symptomatized discontent, armed only with my knowledge of psychiatric labels, and my power to prescribe tricyclics and benzodiazepines.

Doctors and patients

Likewise, when I first became a hospital psychiatrist I felt like a casualty officer in Northern Ireland; I had no idea what all the fighting was about but nevertheless I patched people up, hoped that was sufficient, and sent them on their way.

The following case probably has an all too familiar ring to most psychiatrists and general practitioners, and serves to illustrate some radical questions in contemporary psychiatry.

Patient 1

Mrs B is 30 years of age. She has three children under the age of five years and lives on the 13th floor of a council high-rise block with her husband, who works in a semi-skilled capacity at a car factory. Although the block of flats is only 10 years old, it has the usual stigmata of anonymous public contempt, desecration and fatigued indifference; peeling paintwork, ubiquitous grime, litter and dogs' faeces on the worn floor covering. Aerosoled on the concrete wall outside is an impotent, misspelt, rebellious slogan overtly advertising the National Front, but in reality attempting to purge an uncomfortable burden of blind anger. Mrs B's flat is crowded and has only a small balcony looking out onto a grim, grey, industrial landscape. She spends her day controlling or nurturing her children and either seeing her husband off to work or awaiting his return. The architecture of the flats makes no provision for children to play or mothers to meet, so she sees few other adults during the day. Even shopping is a major expedition because of the demands of her children. Consequently she rarely goes out, and her husband shops at weekends. She welcomes the regular visits by her health visitor if only because it gives her some adult conversation and the opportunity to be looked after for a while when, at almost every other point in her waking life (and sometimes in her dreams as well), she is looking after others.

The health visitor. The health visitor was first allocated to her after the birth of her second child, when she was hospitalized with a 'puerperal depressive illness' and, almost as a matter of routine, was then considered as being 'at risk' with the mothering of her child. In spite of the pleasant and friendly manner of the health visitor, Mrs B feels ambivalent about her. Although she feels she ought to be grateful for the trouble she takes, she perceives dimly that she is being patronised, and that somehow this is irrelevant to her underlying problems, which continue unformulated and unresolved.

Marriage. When Mrs B married at the age of 23 she was impelled largely by romantic fantasies of uncompromised closeness and sharing. Her own parents' relationship had been ground down to a state of indifferent semi-tolerance by their banal and repetitious life, but she did not yet anticipate this for herself. She envisaged her own marriage as plucking her out of this situation, so that her life could become the kind of existence featured in popular women's journals – a state of serene and gratified selflessness earned by courting her family with the whiteness of her wash and lightness of her pastry. The reality has been predictably and bitterly disappointing. Early in their marriage Mr and Mrs B were aware of a sense of emptiness and malaise that they could not articulate, communicate or understand. Mrs B felt emotionally unnourished and discounted, while Mr B felt trapped and nagged at. She needed Valium for her 'anxiety state', and he needed alcohol for his night out with 'the boys'. The birth of their children has driven them even further apart emotionally but, paradoxically, the bonds of guilt between them have grown, so that they both feel doomed to endure their marriage as it is, come what may.

Mr B. Mr B is not an unkind man but is unable to understand what is wrong in his life. Due to his wife's unaccountable (to him) unhappiness, he escapes the endless circular rows at home by saying he has to work late, and finding solace in pubs, male friends and the occasional furtive sexual encounter. Perversely, however, these make things worse rather than better. They both feel increasingly resentful, guilty, inadequate and paranoid, so that their contact together always culminates in a stalemate of alienated conflict. Mr B "just cannot understand it". After all, he works extremely hard and feels he shares the money he earns as fairly as he can. He finds his work as a body-welder monotonous, exhausting and unrewarding. The works milieu is enormous, noisy and anonymous. He repeats the same task about 60 *times daily and, in spite of the increased bargaining power of his union, he continues to feel disposable, unimportant and depersonalized. He has never seen the people who make important policy decisions at his place of work, and his ultimate employers reside in distant boardrooms reified for him only by mediators, memoranda and rumour.*

He is an intelligent man but the deprived background in which he grew up furnished him with neither the norms nor the educational facilities, ever to aspire to further education or professional training. Like so many others in his situation he feels alienated, frustrated and cheated, but is unable to understand the basis of this sensation. His private and stored resentments are sometimes discharged publicly in bargaining disputes, but even when these are resolved with apparent success his underlying sense of oppression remains. He continues to feel trapped and used, but his bills have to be paid and so he works for the money. To counter the industrial wilderness he endures every day, he hopes this year to buy a colour television and spend a couple of weeks in Majorca. Not surprisingly, when he returns home to find a harassed, unhappy and demanding wife, he fails to understand his part in all this. "What more can I do? I work hard and then I get this every evening ... ", he ruminates with glum rhetoric.

Admission to the local psychiatric unit. Their sense of mystified powerlessness is further endorsed by the local psychiatric unit, where Mrs B has been admitted on three occasions in the last five years: twice with a diagnosis of 'puerperal depressive illness', and once with an 'agitated depressive illness'. Both Mr and Mrs B now believe that she has a 'disease of her nerves', which is what her psychiatrist conveyed to them. In any case they both see her unhappy and 'awkward' behaviour at home as being due to her 'depression'. They conceive, vaguely, that Mrs B has a 'fault' inside her and that this, rather than her marital arrangements or the environment in which she must survive, is the root of her difficulties.

Medical assessment. Their general practitioner has also been sucked into this collusion. Like most of us, his training taught him to look at people's problems from a basis of 'illness', from which they could escape only by reliance on medical personnel and their techniques. His view is confirmed by the vast bulk of literature and secondary medical consultations. Consider this letter written to him about Mrs B by the consultant psychiatrist.

"… As you know, Mrs B was admitted here at your request following her increasing depression and agitation, which she had consulted you about in recent weeks. The pattern of this episode was similar to her previous bouts of depression, and was accompanied by early morning wakening and a loss of interest in almost everything, including her appetite. On admission here we found her to be markedly agitated and tearful, with a lot of self-demeaning ideas typical of depression …

"She is a cooperative patient and she made an uneventful recovery on Imipramine 75 mg t.d.s., and a short course of ECT, as she has done previously …

"There is, of course, the question of her children and, in view of her relapsing condition, you will remember that you kindly arranged for a health visitor to visit regularly, and we will try to arrange for one of our nurses to visit. Mr and Mrs B both understand the necessity for this. Mr B seems very supportive, though I understand he works very long hours…

"If she has another relapse it may be worthwhile trying her on Lithium, though I note she had kidney disease as a child. In the meantime she should continue her present dose of Imipramine, and I will see her as an outpatient in three weeks … "

From the phenomenological viewpoint this is a competent medical assessment (except that there is evidence that she recovered from hospitalisation, not medication), but such a style of assessment and care is loaded with politically important assumptions. It conveys authoritatively to Mrs B, and all who are involved with her, that she is the victim of something wrong inside her, that only doctors can understand and alleviate. It conspires with the whole fabric and style of her life in duping her into the belief that she is powerless, and that her world is something she must adjust to, not question or change. There are probably hundreds of thousands of women like Mrs B in the UK today. Theoretically, each one may be viewed as suffering from an affective disorder. From an anthropological view, however, the overall pattern appears more as a concealed form of impotent rebellion and social control, with doctors performing a task similar to, but more technical than, that of policemen.

A radical political view of psychiatry

Awareness of the kind of matrix I have described has led recently to many fundamental and articulate challenges to the present status and ethos of psychiatry. In the USA particularly Radical Psychiatry has a large following. Even those who dismiss their political tenets can still derive perspicacity from the Radical Psychiatrists' clear-headed analysis of the present confused impasse of psychiatry. It is worth noting, however, that not all radical critics of psychiatry are politically left wing. Thomas Szasz is an example.

Claude Steiner, a Radical Psychiatrist in California, started formulating his standpoint at the time of the Vietnam war. This was a time when overt psychiatric morbidity, together with drug abuse among the young, rose to a very high level. The potential abuses and paradoxes of psychiatry became clearly highlighted at this time. Steiner captured this dilemma with a vividness and resolve that arose painfully out of his involvement. He writes:

"Consider a seventeen-year-old American youngster during the Vietnam war. He is told that he must offer his life to destroy the enemy in Asia. He is told that this is good for him, for his brothers and sisters, for his country, and even for the enemy. He is taught that a man will defend his country without question, and that a man who hesitates or questions this principle is a coward who does not deserve to be called a human being. If he fails to understand that he is being oppressed and if he believes these lies, he will eventually come to think of himself as less than human for not wanting to defend his country. He will doubt his own opinions and experiences concerning the war. He will come to consider himself a coward; he will become disgusted with himself; he will cut himself off from his peers and will become depressed. He may lose interest in everyday activities; he may begin to speak about hopelessness and meaninglessness; he may start using drugs to give himself a temporary reprieve from his despair. If his shame and despair reach large enough proportions, he may attempt to destroy himself. He will see himself as no good and will believe himself in need of psychiatric attention.

"If he were to consult a 'neutral' therapist, he might be asked, 'What is wrong with you? Why are you depressed? Why do you hate your father? Why do you rebel against authority? Let's talk about it, and you'll feel better. Tell me about your childhood. Maybe the bad things that happened then make you sad now. Other boys your age aren't depressed about the war and killing. These are troubled times, but others are able to adjust to them. Why don't you? Tell me your dreams. Maybe we can find what is wrong with you. The army is bad, I know, but it has its good points. It might make a man out of you'.

"This young man may eventually feel better because of the friendly and warm attitude of the therapist, thus mystifying his true feelings about the war. He may 'pull himself together', his personality-trait disturbance (passive-aggressive, aggressive type) may improve, and he may wind up in a flag-wrapped box. His therapist will feel and will contend that he was neutral throughout the therapeutic intervention and that he did not attempt to influence the young man. But in truth he acted as a recruiting officer for the army, all the more effective for his disarming smile."

Driven by such experiences, the Radical Psychiatrists drew up their Manifesto, which was presented in 1969 at the Annual Conference of the American Psychiatric Association. Again I quote at length, as I cannot effectively paraphrase:

1. The practice of psychiatry has been usurped by the medical establishment. Political control of its public aspects has been seized by medicine, and the language of soul healing ... has been infiltrated with irrelevant medical concepts and terms.

   "Psychiatry must return to its non-medical origins since most psychiatric conditions are in no way the province of medicine. All persons competent in soul healing should be known as psychiatrists. Psychiatrists should repudiate the use of medically derived words such as 'patient', 'illness', 'diagnosis', 'treatment'. Medical psychiatrists' unique con-tribution to psychiatry is as experts on neurology and, with much needed additional work, on drugs."

2. Extended individual psychotherapy is an elitist, outmoded, as well as non-productive, form of psychiatric help. It concentrates the talents of a few on a few. It silently colludes with the notion that people's difficulties have their sources within them while implying that everything is well with the world. It promotes oppression by shrouding its consequences with shame and secrecy. It further mystifies by attempting to pass as an ideal human relationship when it is, in fact, artificial in the extreme.

"People's troubles have their source not within them, but in their alienated relationships, in their exploitation, in polluted environments, in war, and in the profit motive. Psychiatrists should encourage bilateral, open discussion and discourage secrecy and shame in relation to deviant behaviour and thoughts."

3. By remaining 'neutral' in an oppressive situation, psychiatry, especially in the public sector, has become an enforcer of establishment values and laws. Adjustment to prevailing conditions is the avowed goal of most psychiatric treatment. Persons who deviate from the world's madness are given fraudulent diagnostic tests which generate diagnostic labels which lead to 'treatment' which is, in fact, a series of graded repressive procedures such as 'drug management', hospitalization, shock therapy, perhaps lobotomy. All these forms of 'treatment' are perversions of legitimate medical methods that have been put at the service of the establishment by the medical profession. Treatment is forced on persons who would, if let alone, not seek it.

"Psychological tests and the diagnostic labels they generate, especially schizophrenia, must be disavowed as meaningless mystifications, the real function of which is to distance psychiatrists from people and to insult people into conformity. Medicine must cease making available drugs, hospitals and other legitimate medical procedures for the purpose of overt or subtle law enforcement and must examine how drug companies are dictating treatment procedures through their advertising. Psychiatry must cease playing a part in the oppression of women by refusing to promote adjustment to their oppression. All psychiatric help should be by contract; that is, people should choose when, what, and with whom they want to change. Psychiatrists should become advocates of the people, should refuse to participate in the pacification of the oppressed, and should encourage people's struggles for liberation ..."

An example of radical psychiatric therapy

Patient 2

Mrs E was initially referred to a gynaecologist because of her secondary amenorrhea. He did not feel that her amenorrhea was of great significance, but he became alarmed by her behavioural symptomatology. An urgent psychiatric assessment revealed to me the distressed and bizarre pattern of her present life. Apart from her amenorrhea, she had a marked appetite disturbance, so that she would either starve or gorge herself for periods of weeks, leading to a marked fluctuation in her weight. When gorging herself she would eat packs of butter and sometimes even scraps of food from the dustbin. Her comment about herself during these times was, "I'm fat and gross and disgusting, but I feel so empty; I've got to get something inside me". Her sexual needs were similarly cyclical. When overeating she would be sexually compulsive, insatiable and demanding. When starving herself, her disinclination for sex was so great that she would spend the night in a sleeping bag within her marital bed. In the background was her misery and depression and the 'escape hatch' of recurrently contemplated suicide should things get too bad. Mrs E was not 'acutely ill' insofar as she had received miscellaneous kinds of psychiatric help since a severe marital disruption six years before. Her husband had left her for a few months, leaving behind a trail of lies, veiled threats and innuendoes. She said of that time, "I think I died then. She (the other woman) represented everything I could never be. But it was the lies that hurt me most. Somehow I still think he hates me, although I don't know... ".

It was the custom in the department in which I was working for a committee of psychotherapists to discuss suitability and allocation of all referred cases requiring psychotherapy. They were fascinated but dismayed by what I brought them. Their prevailing view was that her symptomatology represented a severe disturbance, with regression back to an early oral stage of development, with its accompanying psychotic component. Nothing short of extensive individual psychoanalytic psychotherapy, they held, would have any chance of helping her. This would only be possible within the context of private psychoanalysis (which she could afford) or one of the few NHS inpatient psychotherapy units.

Marital problems and family background. By the time the committee's assessment was made, I had a joint interview with Mr and Mrs E. From what I heard and observed, I felt that her overt pathology was quite as much a function of the dynamics of the marriage as Mrs E's intrapsychic difficulties per se. Mrs E had compromised herself for Mr E ever since the beginning of their relationship and, furthermore, her marriage closely resembled her parents'. Early on she supported her husband while he went to art college and, although he had become successful in his work, this pattern had largely continued, so that the bulk of the chores had been carried by Mrs E. She had been oppressed into believing that she was the lesser of the two partners and therefore must subjugate her needs to those of her husband and his work. Her own family had expected her to heed and tend to other people's needs before her own, and she had continued to relate to people in this way. Like many women, she received extremely little gratification for herself directly but was expected to compensate for this by such vicarious gratification as she could eke out of her nurturing role with Mr E and their small son. Ironically, she had come to see both of them in the same light: domineering, demanding and more important and powerful than herself. The resentment and anger that she felt thus came from a thwarted and one-down position. To compound her problems she felt mystified about her feelings, and thus assumed that her 'illness' was due to some fault in her alone.

Therapy. Mr and Mrs E declined the individual psychoanalytic approach that had been suggested and by this time viewed her symptomatology as being a product of their marriage, and had come to *a point of wanting to do something about this. I agreed to work with them with the following explicitly agreed formulations and strategies:*

That Mrs E's 'illness' had arisen because of her muted resentment, and represented her need to have her feelings understood, expressed and cared for. It also signalled her need to have as much space and autonomy as other members of her family.

Much of her sense of passivity arose from the inequality of power in their relationship. Mrs E was either not doing what she wanted, or doing what she did not want, far more often than Mr E.

Her bewilderment had many roots in her husband's mystifying and deceptive behaviour. (Due to his own family background, he had developed a great fear of closeness and a need to 'hide' what was going on in himself.)

Mrs E's part in overcoming these problems was to:
- *clarify for herself what she did and did not want*
- *learn to ask directly for what she wanted*
- *make it clear to Mr E when she was doing anything that she did not want to do*
- *spend a certain amount of time each day doing something that was not at all accountable to others in the family, but was personally gratifying to her.*

Mr E's part was to:
- *really listen to his wife (which involved looking at her)*
- *accept her having her feelings, without trying to parry or rationalise them away*
- *nurture her more, and share much of the domestic work*
- *demystify himself by honestly owning and communicating his thoughts and feelings when she asked him to do so.*

My part in this programme was to remain as impartial as possible, to clarify and interpret, to mediate, to make practical suggestions and to protect them at times of emotional stress. I also undertook to provide alternative medical care if this failed.

Outcome and discussion.

Six months after we had embarked on this contractual therapy, Mrs E was symptomatically clear of her presenting complaints. She spoke with an assurance and warmth that was not evident before. There had been times in therapy where the marriage had looked extremely tenuous, but overall its foundations and communications had become firmer, surer and more equally acknowledged and shared. Most gratifyingly they seemed able to resolve their problems without me.

Such a method of therapy lies outside the medical model and its conventional psychiatric derivatives. Paradoxically, conventional psychiatric therapy ran the risk of driving Mrs E further into the system of thoughts and feelings that was central to her distress. Even classical psychoanalytic psychotherapy would have attempted to label and treat her individually without much emphasis on the real forces that were acting on her in the 'here' and 'now'. The psychoanalytic model would probably formulate her problem as "a narcissistic woman of passive-aggressive type, with weak ego-defences who has regressed or become fixated to an early oral infantile stage, with the mobilization of much archaic and hysterical material. Such material might lead to a psychotic transference reaction in psychotherapy, which should thus be avoided". To Mrs E this would have been as mystifying and alienating as a prescription for Imipramine. More importantly, it would have confirmed for her yet again that there was something wrong with her (although she would never quite understand what 'it' was), that she was powerless, and must continue to be confused in the world in which she found herself.

Acknowledgement

Grateful acknowledgement is made to Grove Press and Claude Steiner for permission to reproduce material from *Readings in Radical Psychiatry.*

Reference

Steiner, C. (ed.), *Readings in Radical Psychiatry,* Grove Press, New York, 1975.

Further reading

Illich, I., *The Medical Nemesis,* Calder and Boyars, London, 1974.

Steiner, C. *Scripts People Live,* Grove Press, New York, 1974.

Szasz, T. *The Myth of Mental Illness,* Paladin, London, 1972.

Szasz, T, *Ideology and Insanity,* Calder and Boyars, London, 1973.

Szasz, T. *The Manufacture of Madness,* Routledge and Kagan Paul, London, 1971.

Wycoff, H. Love, *Therapy and Politics,* Grove Press. New York, 1976.

Published in *Update* 1978, 105

The Elements of Psychotherapy

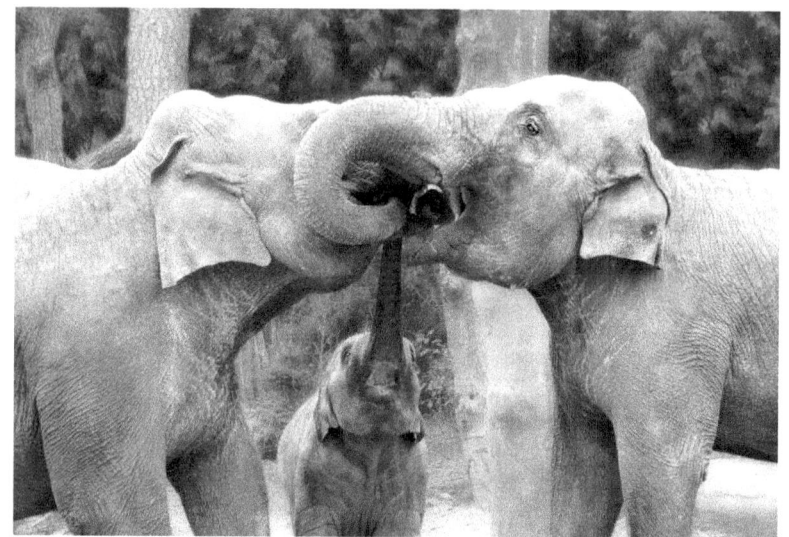

'… Much will be gained if we succeed in transforming your hysterical misery into common unhappiness. With a mental life that has been restored to health, you will be better armed against that unhappiness.'

(Freud, 1895, *Studies on Hysteria*).

Psychotherapy is a subtle activity, often opaque to outsiders. One definition might be: it is the deliberate and structured use of a professional relationship, enabling an individual to explore, discover and express aspects of themselves that otherwise would remain hidden and troublesome. Certain things follow: this expanded awareness and expressivity can then bring about a fuller, freer, better adapted self and its relationship with others. Put another way, psychotherapy is getting help to understand and express oneself more clearly and fully, so that we are empowered to grow beyond self-limiting or self-defeating patterns. Liberation from such internal traps and tangles, enables us to make choices that are more realistically gratifying and creatively responsive.

These definitions, although probably acceptable to most psychotherapists, are likely to arouse either confusion or scepticism in many medical practitioners. Pragmatically, what can it achieve, and how? When is it most likely to work, and in which form? What is its relevance to medical practice? This article offers some introductory answers to these questions.

Psychopathology

Before the elements of psychotherapy can be understood, it is necessary to survey some of the principles of 'psychopathology': the theory of what goes wrong for individuals, and why.

The basics of these are:
- As infants and small children we are all highly vulnerable, in much need of attention and protection. We probably have a rich, sometimes violent fantasy life, and are unable for some

years to subject this to reality-testing (Bowlby, 1971, 1975, 1981; Klein, quoted in Segal, 1964; Piaget, 1952).

• It follows that the infant and young child are crucially dependent on caring figures for stability, safety, reality-testing and love. Consequently, if these are not forthcoming, the person will grow up with an impairment of his image of self and others. These determine our ability to relate trustingly, realistically and positively; to develop our own creativity and to healthily integrate our most primitive impulses or feelings (Bowlby, 1971, 1975, 1981; Balint, 1968; Winnicott, 1965). The latter requires an inwardly directed capacity for reality-testing (Rosen, 1962; Schiff, 1975).

• Some feelings and impulses are very threatening to the conscious self and its sense of integrity. This may lead to 'ego-defence mechanisms', which are involuntary attempts to ward off destabilising internal conflict or distress (Freud, 1936). When excessive, these defence mechanisms may themselves cause problems: 'presenting symptoms', ranging from recurrent relationship difficulties to mental and physical illness (Freud, 1963).

• In suitable and motivated individuals, such dysfunctional patterns may be ameliorated or resolved by professional help. This happens by:

• Perceiving and understanding the origin and current consequences of such patterns. This is a large part of historical *insight*.

• Experiencing, within the therapeutic relationship, an encouragement, consistency or caring which was lacking in early original experiences. This can enable *healing*.

• Acknowledging, experiencing and expressing feelings and impulses that have become fearsome and forbidden for the individual. This unlocking can free the individual for *growth*.

• Recognizing the distinction between archaic yearnings, frustrations and impulses, and present reality. This kind of operational insight will help an individual navigate the lifelong psychological tasks of *immunity, growth* and *repair* (Perls *et al.*, 1973; Berne, 1961).

The tool of talking

It is sometimes claimed, particularly by those whose outlook is mechanistic, that 'talking can't do any good', or 'you can't change a person's make-up'. In a sense these claims are true, in that words cannot have the same predictable impact on another person, as can a surgical procedure or a drug when the doctor necessarily assumes control over the patient's internal processes. Physical medical treatment is unilateral and hence more controllable than the bilateral process of psychotherapy, where the *dialogue* is at the very centre of its effect. The patient is here far from being a passive recipient; he is an active synthesizer, and ultimately the effectiveness of what is given depends on what he does with it.

Given these limitations, verbal communication can still be immensely valuable when used skilfully and appositely. Its benefits are various and multiple. It can be an antidote to isolation, a way of externalizing internal confusion and thus gaining clarity or a different perspective, a method of de-pressurizing built-up feeling systems and – perhaps most important – a way of forming a *common language* with another person. This latter is an important step to creating a compassionate understanding and acceptance, both of the self and others. Such a common language can only develop, however, when there is a *therapeutic rapport*: this itself implies the conscious wish to develop capacities for trust, discovery and sharing. Some aspects involved in this process are depicted in figure 1 (Luft, 1966).

	Known to self	Unknown to self
Known to others	Public self ①	Blind self ②
Unknown to others	Secret self ③	Unconscious self ④

FIG. 1.—*Operational parts of the self*

It can be seen that different styles or levels of psychotherapy can act to bring about different kinds of integration of parts of the self:

A depressed and isolated man, unhappy with his loneliness, is unaware of the way he is critical of those who approach him. Other members of a therapy group confront him with this, and he begins to see his contribution to his problem. *Integration of (1) and(2).*

A woman who is ambivalent about her sexual relationships begins tentatively to talk to her therapist about the misty but intense sexual longings she used to have for her father, about which she still feels guilty and afraid. *Integration of (3) and(1).*

A middle-aged man, prone to depressive episodes when he feels rejected, tells of a dream, which the therapist thinks indicates his lifelong searching for his father who died when the patient was a boy; the patient denied missing or thinking about him much prior to the dream. *Integration of (4) and (3) and (1).*

Why do we need to integrate these different parts? In general it can be said that:

It is not possible to have mastery of those parts of ourselves of which we are unaware.

Relegating distressing and unresolved parts of ourselves to secrecy is likely to seriously limit our capacity for intimate and authentic attachments, and may 'leak out' to produce symptoms.

It is only possible to be competent and responsive social beings if we have a fairly clear idea of how other people see us.

Of course, the mere awareness, or expression, of these unintegrated parts of the self does not of itself bring about the required change or integration, but they are essential prerequisites. In much the same way, a map may help us plan a journey, but it cannot bring about the travelling for us. The actual 'travelling' in psychotherapy is a complex matter, involving many different components of resource and motivation, in both patient and therapist.

Almost all psychotherapeutic interventions are some type of *support*, *confrontation* or *interpretation*. Each of these may be a powerful facilitator when used correctly, but may be damaging when untimely or poorly attuned.

Figure 2 – *The therapeutic triad*

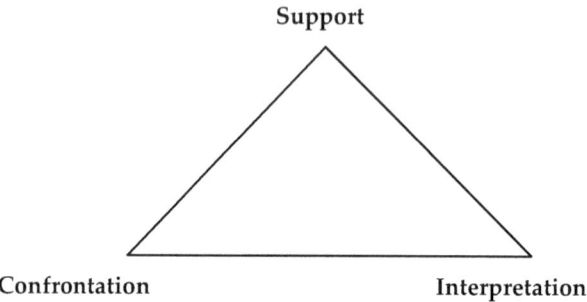

Support

Support interventions are those that accept the patient as he is, without the pressure for greater awareness or change. It creates what Winnicott (1965) termed 'the facilitating environment'; a *safe base* from which the patient may begin the more difficult task of exploring and expressing material which has not previously been verbalized or shared. It is a paradox of the human condition that often we cannot change the way we operate until we have really accepted ourselves as we are. As a consequence, the therapist must at first accept the patient as he is and support him in his present *modus vivendi,* before other endeavours are undertaken. For this reason many therapists would agree that skilful support is the most basic element in this triad; often, an individual will find his own resources and understanding merely with such help. This is particularly true of those reacting immediately to loss and other crises, and thus is particularly pertinent to the work of the general practitioner. The style of therapy derived from Carl Rogers (1961) and counselling holds that 'unconditional positive regard' is the most important facilitator in therapy. However, for more severe difficulties such as prolonged grief reactions, or longstanding personality disturbance, a therapy with other components of the triad is called for.

Interpretation

Interpretation helps a patient to make new sense of communicated experience by deliberately introducing associations with previously unlinked experiences and images. In general, it is true to say that there are no 'right' or 'wrong' interpretations, only those that a patient can use within the therapeutic rapport. Thus, an interpretation that may be 'correct' to the therapist but cannot be assimilated by the patient is edifying only to the former and, if asserted dogmatically, will damage the development of rapport. In this sense interpretations should not be 'made' or 'given', but 'offered' tentatively and experimentally. When interpretations are successful they lead to a *deepening of rapport* (Malan, 1979), where the patient feels an increase both in his own understanding and the sense of his being understood, so that he feels safe to explore and share more (Menninger, 1958). Often the most gratifying and facilitating examples of interpretation are also the simplest.

The following two examples illustrate some of these principles:

Example 1

A young woman had been admitted to hospital four times in five years with episodes of mania. Her treatment had consisted mainly of custody and suppression of her symptoms with drugs, evidently with limited and transient effect. On her last admission she exhibited her usual pattern of grandiose thinking and hyperactivity, but the doctor was aware of her eyes glistening. After spending a while with her, he said gently: 'underneath all this activity and bravado, I get the sense that really you're feeling very sad and helpless'. She collapsed and sobbed for several minutes, confirming the doctor's intuition of concealed feelings underlying her 'manic defence'. Later, albeit with pain and difficulty, she developed a sufficient therapeutic alliance with the doctor to explore some of the unarticulated emotional problems generating her episodic illness.

Example 2

A woman in her early forties was convicted of a shoplifting offence and referred for psychotherapy. Six months before her offence she had had a hysterectomy. She was late for her initial interview and the male therapist found her to be 'sexually provocative'; he then made an interpretation to the effect that she had wanted to redress her sexual loss by stealing, first from the shop, and now from him (his time and his penis). She curtly denied understanding of either the remark or its relevance, and did not attend further appointments.

This complex interpretation may have been psychoanalytically 'correct', but was untimely and unwieldy: it could not be incorporated into the fragile rapport between patient and therapist, which had only just begun. This woman did not feel sufficiently understood and accepted as she was to be able to use such a comment, which was experienced by her as an attack or derogation.

Confrontation

Confrontation is a term used to describe the therapist's action when he directly draws attention to an aspect of a patient's behaviour, without offering an explanation. Its aim is to enhance *awareness* of behaviour; the way in which he operates and how this may affect others. Generally, attention is focused on what is currently happening. Therefore group and family therapy often utilise this type of intervention because of the richness of interplay between its members, who will act as both confronter and confronted. The therapist's role is then to keep the confrontation within a scope of intensity and relevance that will be tolerable and therapeutic. If a patient is to consider seriously and assimilate the subject of confrontation, he must first feel an adequate sense of care and safety in the therapeutic setting, otherwise he will merely feel attacked. This will lead to an escalation of his defences, rather than the reverse.

Example 3

A middle-aged man complained bitterly and with hurt about his estrangement from his son, who he described as secretive and surly. The therapist noticed his own sense of irritation and exasperation with the patient, who continually, but without apparent awareness, talked across the therapist, and made inaccurate assumptions about him. The therapist gently but firmly pointed this out, adding that this pattern was possibly also true with the son, leading to the painful impasse he had described. Because the man had a trusting rapport with the therapist, he was able to acknowledge and explore this pattern.

Confrontation is a prominent component of the newer, humanistic therapies such as Encounter, Gestalt and Transactional Analysis. These can be potent catalysts to awareness of present functioning. However, this potency has the capacity to harm, by engendering too much material too quickly for the patient to handle. This caveat leads to the 'Rule of the Therapeutic Triad', which may be stated as: 'For rapport in psychotherapy to be maintained and beneficial, interpretation or confrontation should not exceed the support that is offered to the patient'.

Transference

It has already been outlined how our internal world-image and self-image is fundamentally influenced by our early experiences. All of us, more or less consciously, act from and act-out the kind of adjustments and decisions we made in infancy and early childhood. It follows that we transfer onto others our expectations and fears deriving from that period. If these early experiences were generally good and satisfactorily resolved, this will lead to healthy growth and adjustment. For those who were not so fortunate, the result will be recurrent and continuing difficulties with relationships, and expression and gratification of the self. In such cases it is important that the patient is able to understand what he is *projecting* onto others that hampers him, so that he may be able to grow beyond these ancient repetitions. This field of archaic projections is termed *transference* in psychotherapy and, in the more analytic therapies, is considered the most important diagnostic and therapeutic tool. In these 'deeper' therapies, it is thought to be necessary for the patient to:

Experience, in the present, the kind of fears, expectations and fantasies he had as a child and which he now projects onto the therapist (*Evolution* of transference).

With the help of the therapist, to understand their historical roots and present way of operating (*Analysis* of transference).

Slowly abandon these methods of functioning, by finding newer and more productive ways of relating to the therapist (*Resolution* of transference).

The analysis, or interpretation, of transference may be depicted by another triangle.

Figure 3. *The triangle of transference*

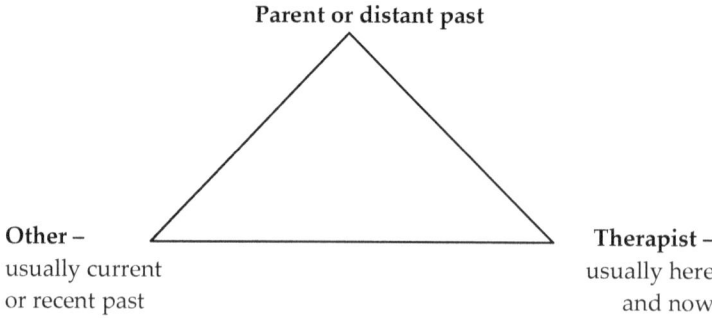

Figure 3 illustrates a scheme whereby the influence of the past may be understood in terms of both the therapy and the patient's current life-situation. For the fullest understanding, links are perceived between all three; at other times more partial insight may be gained by linking any two of the three.

Example 3 (continued)

After the middle-aged man understood how he was warding off the therapist, he began to see how he was also doing this with his son (O-T link). The therapist then asked him how he felt when he behaved like this, and then whether he could remember this same feeling when he was very young. The patient then became eager to talk about his fear of domination by others — even his son — and how he attempted to counter this by pre-empting and defining others. He then went on to talk of his relationship with his father and older brother, who he felt exerted a bullying alliance against him. He talked of his recurrent feelings of fear, humiliation and resentment. From this account he began to see how his experiences of the past were being re-enacted both with his son and the therapist (O-P and O-T links), and began to feel less bewildered and powerless in the face of his feelings.

Applicability of psychotherapy

Psychotherapy in its different forms may be helpful for a wide spectrum of disturbance or distress: from disabling life-crises, to chronically unsatisfactory patterns of adjustment or relationships. Always, though, the following are essential for any success:

• That the individual recognizes that he is not merely a victim of circumstances or faulty biological mechanism, but that he, in some way, is now an *active agent* in his pattern of distress.

• That he is willing, at least consciously, to pursue the possibility that reflecting on himself and sharing himself, in a professional setting, may lead to a newer and more worthwhile kind of integration and understanding. This is a complex issue, as there are frequently unconscious forces working against conscious motivation – the patient's 'resistance' – when, paradoxically, the distressed mode of functioning is equated with familiarity and security, and is therefore resistant to real examination or change.

• The patient must be able and willing to tolerate the frustration and pain that often accompanies 'the therapeutic process'. Self-disclosure and acknowledgement of long-buried parts of the self is often difficult and requires considerable investment and courage. It is here that the skill and personal qualities of the therapist can ameliorate the situation. It is also important that the patient understands the metaphorical nature of the relationship; for the care and attention he receives, and the feelings or impulses he has toward the therapist, are at the same time authentic but ritualized within the framework and boundaries of the setting. The patient must have the intent and capacity to 'talk-out', and not 'act-out', his difficulties.

It is the therapist's empathic and professional skills that can elicit, maintain and guide these capacities in the patient. When this happens, there is said to be a strong *therapeutic alliance* between patient and therapist, and they may create a *common language* that unifies the patient's experience of himself and the therapist's experience and understanding of him. The ability to pursue this at the beginning of therapy is usually a favourable prognostic sign, and also indicates the formation of a safe-base from which the patient may experience and work out his 'negative transference' towards the therapist – his covert and archaic fear, envy, anger or resentment – which may underlie his inability to make trusting or intimate relationships.

Many authors have drawn attention to the caution that should be applied in using psychotherapy in those suffering from severe mental illness, such as psychotic or obsessive-compulsive syndromes, or in personalities with poor social control. It is probably true, however, that these criteria apply equally to these more disabled people, as to the more common (and more easily identified-with) neurotic (Rosen, 1962); that, if a therapeutic alliance can be forged and a common language created (that requires special skill and experience), then the patient may grow away from his disturbed impasse.

Psychotherapy and medicine

Psychotherapy and medicine work from very different assumptions: the former works from the position that the patient must develop his own resources, clarification and self-definition, while the medical model works from the opposite pole; the doctor provides the resources (treatment) and definition (diagnosis). The medical patient may present the problem, but it is soon converted into the language of the doctor who then commands the dialogue (Zigmond, 1982). Psychotherapy, in searching for a common language, cannot therefore be so rigidly defined in its process or outcome; because it has its roots in personal and evolving dialogue, it cannot be 'given' or 'prescribed', and it is probably fundamentally misleading to refer to it as a 'treatment': this word usually implies a passive patient who is cured by an active doctor.

In spite of these apparent incongruities, psychotherapeutic insight and technique has a definite place in helping the medical doctor to understand his own and the patient's behaviour and the meaning of patients' symptoms, particularly when these are not readily diagnosed and treated by conventional means (Zigmond, 1977; Balint, 1956). There are evident limits as to how much psychotherapy a doctor can competently and ethically introduce into his medical practice; he would be unwise, for example, to attempt to help a patient with recurrent relationship difficulties to work through primitive anxieties and conflicts, although exceptionally this is possible. He is, however, well-placed to recognize his patient's anxieties and help him to verbalize them, which is, in itself, often perceived by the patient as an act of great understanding and comfort. This is particularly so at times of crisis and loss, as the following example illustrates.

Example 4

A 70-year-old man, Mr F, consulted his doctor, complaining that he woke at night 'feeling like my body is on fire, and I get this terrible itching all over, so that I just can't stop scratching'. Routine physical examination and questioning confirmed that the cause was most unlikely to be organic, and the doctor explained this. The doctor, in simple terms, went on to explain that sometimes it is difficult to express or resolve certain kinds of feelings and thoughts. These then upset the body, causing the kind of symptoms of which Mr F complained. The doctor asked Mr F if this made any sense to him and, if so, whether he had any idea of the kind of thoughts and feelings that were troubling him. Mr F replied that his trouble had started soon after his wife had died, of cancer, three months previously, and he wondered if this had anything to do with it. The doctor maintained a warm and attentive silence, which encouraged Mr F to say, 'It's stupid, I know, to be so upset after this time; I should be over it by now', which the doctor softly countered by reassuring him that such a basic loss often leaves a very long wake of disturbed feelings – that none of us ever completely leaves behind the hurt or the sadness from such a loss. At this point Mr F cried, and then talked about his sense of emptiness, and also his hidden regrets. The doctor then asked him if he was also angry that his wife had been taken away, or had abandoned him, leaving him alone – that although it is not 'rational', all of us can feel angry when we lose someone precious. Yes, Mr F agreed, he had at first been angry with the hospital, then himself, for her death; he knew it didn't make sense, but he still felt resentful. The doctor asked if he had talked with anyone about these feelings; 'No, doctor, not like this. People have their own lives to lead. I don't like to bother them'.

After another few minutes Mr F could see that his feelings were inevitable and important; they could only be conjured out of mind by the development of disturbance elsewhere, i.e. his skin. He found, too, that he could begin to share his feelings; his parting remark was simple but deeply felt: 'Thank you so much for listening to me, doctor. It's good to know there's somebody who understands how I feel'.

Comment: integrating the elements of psychotherapy

The example of Mr F illustrates how some of the elements of psychotherapy may be brought to bear in situations other than intensive psychotherapy programmes. He represented a problem familiar to many doctors who attempt to provide some form of holistic care, and it is arguable that such basic psychotherapeutic skills should be part of their clinical repertoire.

Mr F did not need the kind of prolonged psychotherapy required to help longstanding personality or relationship difficulties, but rather psychotherapeutically enlightened practice. The doctor first of all created a situation, a 'facilitating environment', where a therapeutic alliance evolved. Mr F felt sufficiently supported and trusting to reveal his 'secret self'. The doctor had then gone on to interpret his somatic defence, which enabled Mr F to share his underlying grief and resentment. Because the doctor had shown care and understanding to the vulnerable part of Mr F, the lonely widower would now probably adopt a more tolerant and understanding attitude to his own 'unreasonable' feelings This acceptance could then free him, to heal and find a new equilibrium. It is also important that the doctor was prudent in the use of his interpretations; he refrained from attempting to explore the patient's deeper unconscious where, perhaps, there had been hostile feelings to his wife when she was alive, and for which he now felt guilty. If this were true, it would become manifest later, and to raise this issue in an untimely and premature way would do more harm than good; it would seriously undermine their nascent therapeutic alliance. In this respect one of the most important elements of psychotherapy, as in medicine, is knowing when and where to stop.

$$\Omega$$

References

Balint, M. (1956) *The Doctor, His Patient and the Illness* Pitman, London.
Balint, M. (1968) *The Basic Fault.* Tavistock, London.
Berne, E. (1961) *Transactional Analysis in Psychotherapy* Evergreen, New York.
Bowlby, J. (1971, 1975, 1981) *Attachment and Loss, Vols. 1, 2 and 3.* Hogarth Press, London.
Freud, A. (1936) *The Ego and Mechanisms of Defence* Hogarth Press, London.
Freud, S. (1963) *The Complete Psychological Works. Vols. 15 and 16.* Hogarth Press, London.
Luft, J. (1966) *Group Processes: An Introduction to Group Dynamics* Palo Alto National Press, Palo Alto.
Malan, D. H. (1979) *Individual Psychotherapy and the Science of Psychodynamic* Butterworth, Sevenoaks.
Menninger, K. (1958) *The Theory of Psychoanalytic Technique* Basic Books, New York.
Perls, F., Hefferline, R.F. and Goodman, P. (1973) *Gestalt Therapy* Penguin, London.
Piaget, J. (1952) *The Origins of Intelligence in Children* New York International Universities Press, New York.
Rogers, C.R. (1961) *Client Centred Therapy* Houghton Mifflin, Boston.
Rosen, J. (1962) *Direct Psychoanalytic Psychiatry* Grune and Strattas, New York.
Schiff, J. (1975) *Cathexis Reader* Harper and Row, New York.
Segal. H. (1964) *An introduction to the Work of Melanie Klein* Heinemann. London.
Winnicott, D. W. (1965) *The Maturational Process and the Facilitating Environment* Hogarth Press, London.

Zigmond, D. (1982) *The Psychosomatic Approach* April: 699-709

Zigmond, D. *The Psychosomatic Mosaic* The Practitioner, April: 711-720

Zigmond, D. (1977) *Scientific Psychiatry: Progress or Regress?* Update, October: 675-679

Further reading

Brown, D. and Pedder, J. (1979) *Introduction to Psychotherapy* Tavistock, London.

Kovel, J. (1976) *A Complete Guide to Therapy* Pantheon.

Storr, A. (1979) *The Art of Psychotherapy* Heinemann Medical. London.

Publ. in The Practitioner 1280, *Psychopathology* Vol. 225, Sept. 1981

A Psychosomatic Approach

'I have never yet seen a case of psychological ulcerative colitis!'

A physician's retort to a psychiatrist at a case conference

The very term 'psychosomatic' produces difficulties. It attempts to capture patterns of physical distress or dysfunction which are not simply caused by physical determinants. The structure of the word itself indicates an outlook in which mind and body are considered *together*. However, Western theory and practice of medicine is so thoroughly rooted in Newtonian scientific thought, a system which we rarely question, that the psychosomatic approach continues to evoke mystification, confusion and denial. The foregoing quotation perhaps typifies these reactions in a doctor adopting a defensive attitude to a psychosomatic viewpoint. This series of two articles explores and clarifies some basics of the psychosomatic approach; they are not intended to be authoritative statements on the subject. They offer an outline as to how different kinds of medical practice tackle this problem, and how both patients and doctors perceive, and act upon, different parts of this problem at different times.

The somatic approach

To understand our difficulties with the psychosomatic* viewpoint, we need first to survey briefly the roots and assumptions of our present medical practice. Medicine and medical psychiatry are based on the disciplines of the (Newtonian) physical sciences and their underlying philosophies of dualism and determinism. Dualism, explicated in the writing of Descartes, Malebranche and Geulinx (Russell, 1961), holds that the world is composed of two separate substances, matter and mind, which are independent but synchronous in activity; the two modes are governed by their own laws and run parallel courses (fig. 1).

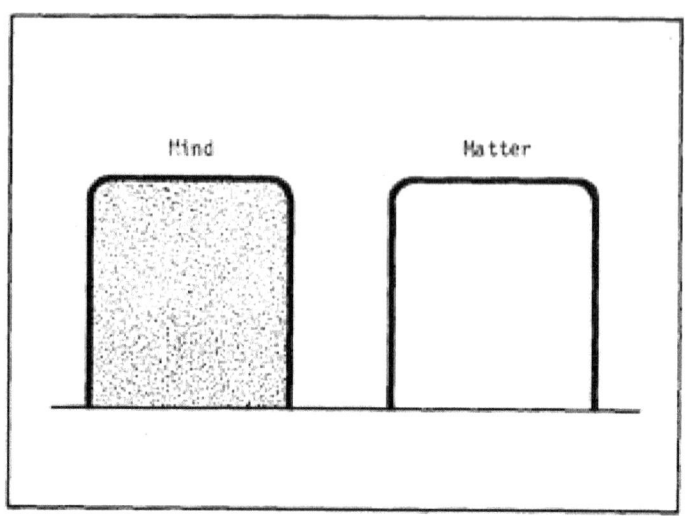

FIG. I.—*Philosophical dualism. Mind and matter separate.*

Newtonian physics, and the consequent school of scientific determinism, takes these assumptions ever further. There is an axiom here that only outwardly observable events (matter) are valid and `real'. Mind or experience are subsumed under the dictates and laws of this observable world in such a way that the subjective world ceases to be of importance, and is regarded as an artefact or interference.

This scientific determinism is the root and prevalent philosophy in our present Western technological culture, where the bulk of our endeavours incline to engineering, that is, the direct alteration and control of physical structures. Medical practice, deriving from this outlook, is based on the assumption that distress can only be alleviated by changing behavioural or physical manifestations of that distress. Antacids for dyspepsia, tranquillizers for anxiety, and behaviour therapy for sexual dysfunction are clinical examples of this engineering philosophy. The experience of distress, it is held, will yield to control of its physical determinants; there is no need to explore or amplify the experience itself, as the experience is only a reflection of disturbed underlying mechanism.

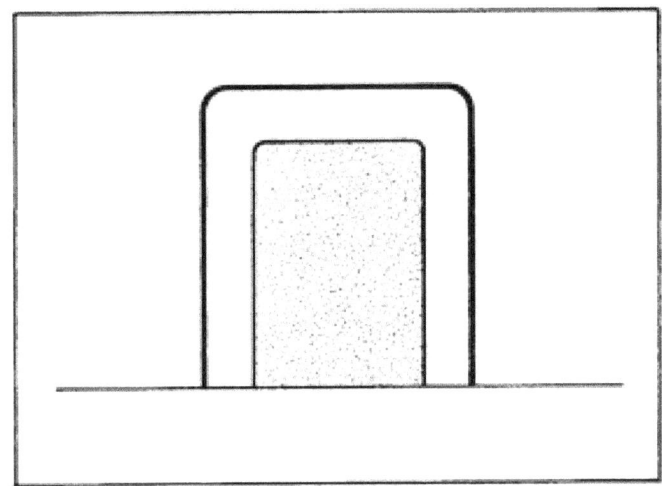

FIG. 2 — Scientific determinism. Matter determines mind (somatic approach).

In clinical practice this approach may be termed 'somatic', and an essential component of this system is the concept of physical causation (fig.2). This defines events as being hierarchical in operation, so that one happening is rigidly determined by its material antecedent. Such a somatic-causational frame of reference is highly effective, even mandatory, in certain clinical situations; for example, when attending the patient with a perforated duodenal ulcer. At other times, however, it may be simplistic to the point of exclusion and distortion.

An example of this might be the unhappy asthmatic child whose disease is said to be caused by house-dust mite allergy; even if the allergy is dealt with, he may still remain wheezy. And then if the wheezing is controlled, he may well succumb to some other form of illness. Such problems are common in primary medical care, when simple physical diagnoses are evidently inadequate to explain the patient who suffers from a changing mosaic of apparently unrelated complaints, or the family which seems prone to perennial illness (Balint, 1957).

Monism

What is lacking in the latter situation is a *holistic* approach that deals with the person, his experiences and environment in a less piecemeal, and more global, manner. Philosophically this alternative approach has been termed 'monism' and is represented in our culture by the philosophical writings of Spinoza and Bergson. Here there is no division of the world into mind and matter; there is only one substance which is experienced differently: internally as mind and externally as matter (fig. 3). The differences are due to the different positions of those undergoing the experiences, not the nature of events *per se*.

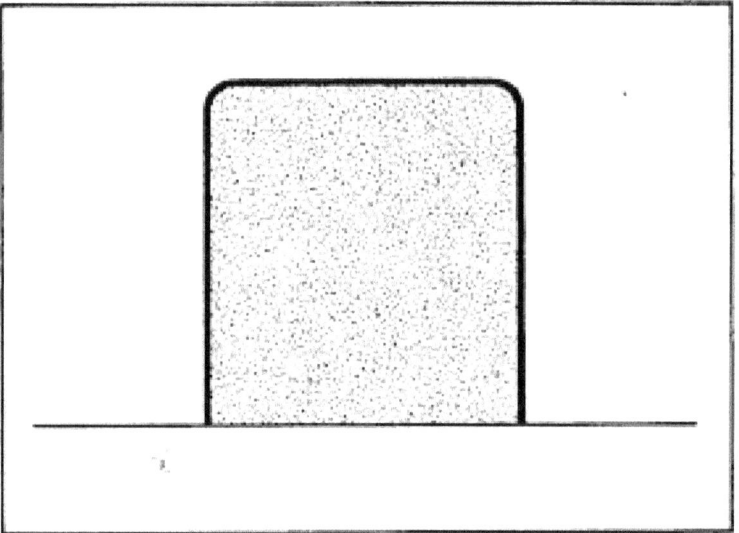

FIG. 3.—*Monism or holism. Matter-mind coexistent and indivisible (Psychosomatic approach).*

It is sometimes claimed that such an approach is unscientific but, in fact, it accords with the development of physics since Heisenberg (Russell, 1959) and Einstein (Einstein and Infeld, 1938). Relativity physics, for example, demonstrates that events and structures which appear to have a definite order or design to one observer, will show a different pattern to a differently placed observer. Consequently, the concept of causation breaks down, as one event does not necessarily precede another unless the frames of reference of the observers are similar. Physics overcomes this by fusing space and time which were previously conceived as inviolable and distinct. By analogy, a holistic approach integrates mind and body in the same way that relativity physics has fused space and time.

Within this model it can be seen that there is not a simple causational (hierarchical) relationship between mind and body; they are merely different aspects of the organism. A change in the body is bound to be accompanied by a shift in mental equilibrium and vice versa. The two are co-existent and indivisible. While the deterministic approach looks for a causal relationship between mind and body, the holistic approach observes changes in the whole organism. An example of this can be illustrated by the two different views on an anxious person with ulcerative colitis. The somatic approach will conceive of the anxiety and colonic inflammation as being 'caused by' disturbances in neurotransmitters, inflammatory mediators etc. The psychosomatic approach will view the experience of anxiety and the signs of colitis as being manifestations of disturbance within the whole person and his environmental field; the inflamed colon and the experience of anxiety being the small part of the disturbance, which both patient and doctor are aware of at the present time.

There are important theoretical and practical difficulties which arise from the traditional scientific method, and what can be contained within it. In the world of biology, science, as elsewhere, is confined to the outward and material manifestations of life. The inner experience, or mind, remains unobserved and thus outside strict scientific assessment of formulation. The nearest that such methods can get to the mind is through such signals as words and behaviour, from which we assume the inner experience. It follows that the somatic approach fits most comfortably within the scientific compass, while the psychosomatic method flows outside in many directions. The validity of the psychosomatic framework is, therefore, difficult to appraise objectively; as I shall suggest in the next article, it may only be practically effective if it has subjective meaning, particularly where the patient is concerned. This may account for the many confusingly inconclusive or negative studies which have been scientifically designed to discern components of 'anxiety' or 'depression' in illness, or the efficacy of psychotherapy in their relief. In these studies the unmeasurable variables are subtle and possibly innumerable, so that studies of complex clinical problems necessarily reduce them to a somatic distillate; the truly psychological (experiential) component having evaporated in the process.

It is crucial to note that there is no 'right' or `wrong' approach. By analogy, relativity physics has not indiscriminately supplanted Newtonian physics. The two systems have different areas of operation and different yields. Sometimes the somatic approach is entirely satisfactory for the task at hand, at other times the psychosomatic approach will be more effective. Inappropriate use of the somatic approach leads to practice that is too simplified, unnecessarily intrusive or controlling, and alienating. On the other hand, when the psychosomatic approach is used indiscriminately it can lead to practice that is dangerously unfocused or inactive. It will be indicated later how there are often subtle factors of dependency, both in the patient and his doctor, which largely decide which kind of model is used in any particular medical situation.

East and West

At this point it is interesting to observe that different cultures have traditionally conceived the world differently, leading to contrasting types of medical practice. The West, which is increasingly influenced by a materialist-determinist philosophy and its consequent technology, has produced a pattern of medical practice which is strongly somatic in its bias; we consume an ever-increasing quantity of drugs to allay our discomfort or distress. Grief, despair, madness, or sexual disinclination, are all easily slotted into syndromes for which a prescription is found. The pursuit of the `biochemical cause' of, for example, cancer and schizophrenia is to our technological culture what the Holy Grail was to early Christian societies. The results of such endeavours are often not dissimilar. Eastern and pre-industrial cultures are traditionally more monistic or psychosomatic in their approach; mind and body are not analytically dislocated as they are in the West. It is believed, therefore, that any attention to the body will change the mind, while calming the mind is bound to reduce disturbance in the body. The repertoire of resulting practices, which is extremely varied and often incomprehensible to those of us familiar only with Western practice, includes massage, yoga, incantation, exorcism, dietary rituals and acupuncture. At present many people are turning to these Eastern practices, which may reflect a disillusionment with the overgrowth of our medical technology and other cultural trends, experienced as controlling and depersonalising (Illich, 1976).

Even the world of non-organic psychiatry is subject to this division. Traditional Western therapies evolved from a scientific-deterministic framework. Psychoanalysis, ultimately has its roots in Freud's training as a neurologist, and behaviour therapy is based on learning theory. In both of these, the model of disturbance and therapy incorporates the notion of a determining cause. Also, they tend to be applied within a highly defined mode of experience; the latter with overt behaviour patterns, the former with verbal communications. Some of the new humanistic therapies have attempted to incorporate Eastern monism. Gestalt (Perls *et al*, 1951) and bioenergetic therapy (Lowen, 1976), for example, regard bodily and mental experiences as being correlative and interchangeable. In these therapies there is equal attention paid to all forms of experience, sensation and behaviour. It is noteworthy, also, that the former types of therapy have found a place in the current realm of medical practice, while the latter have not yet found a comparable assimilation.

The responsibility spectrum

Illness, as usually conceived, is separate from the self as experienced in our conscious thoughts and feelings. It is something that 'happens to', or 'attacks', the self through organisms, accidents or fate. It is not usually considered as the expression or function of the self. The complex of intention, thought and feeling (the self) is thought to be quite different from the world of the body, much as a person and the house he lives in are thought to be distinct. This, of course, is the dualistic approach.

The doctor's conception of illness, and its relationship to the self, often veers even further towards the scientific-deterministic view, which sees a person as being controlled and defined by his body through genetics, chemical transmitters and the like. The quintessence of this approach is found in 'organic psychiatry', which considers mental and behavioural aspects of a person to be 'caused' by an underlying physical matrix. The fact that this matrix is often not well substantiated or defined does not detract from the influence of this model in practice (Zigmond, 1977).

It can be seen that these two approaches see illness as 'ego-dystonic', that is, having no connection with conscious volition, feeling or responsibility of the self. Illness becomes a fault in the machinery of the body; such mechanisms being dictated by the impersonal forces of physics and chemistry. The person is merely a passive and powerless onlooker to his internal processes. Changing such processes, if possible, is seen as coming from the outside, through powerful agencies which manipulate the physical and chemical mechanisms. Alleviation of illness thus becomes the responsibility of the medical attendant, not the patient. When a person goes to a doctor as a patient he largely disowns and encapsulates his distressing experience, and expects the doctor to define it and take it away (Zigmond, 1977). Often, of course, this system is efficient and mandatory; a man with renal colic cannot be expected to make his own diagnosis and relieve his own pain. At other times, however, the issue is less clear-cut. Perhaps most primary medical consultations do not involve structural disease, but rather disturbances of function and bodily experience, which are related to conflicting and unexpressed feeling. Tension headaches, 'needing a tonic', nonspecific musculoskeletal and abdominal discomforts make up a large part, if not the bulk, of the primary doctor's work. Such complaints sometimes yield to suggestion and physical intervention alone. More often, however, this application of the Medical Model serves only to parry the distress syndrome for short periods of time. My next article will explore how application of other non-deterministic models may make more substantial therapeutic inroads into these clinical situations.

If a person's distress is conceived by that person as an expression of inner conflict or turmoil, he is unlikely to think of himself as ill, merely distressed. In this instance the complaint is 'ego-syntonic' ; the bodily disturbance and the self are perceived as a unit. The sufferer sees his experience as being his own responsibility; he may wish that someone (for instance a doctor) could assume responsibility for taking away his discomfort, but in reality he knows that this is not possible. If such a person asks for help it is for compassion, suggestions or new understanding, not magical exorcism. Naturally, it is uncommon for a person to contact his doctor from the outset with these notions, although he may acquire them through consultation.

Such a process of identification is called 'gaining insight', and marks a shift in the patient's thought and feeling process, from a dualistic/deterministic to a monistic/holistic approach to his distress. This change implies also a shift in ownership and responsibility of distress from the doctor back to the patient. It is an important intention of psychotherapy for psychosomatic complaints; in this area the aim of psychotherapy is to help the patient 'identify with' his symptoms so that they are seen as a reflection of feelings, needs or conflicts that are not being dealt with successfully in other ways. Such holistic awareness confers a personal and creative meaning on symptoms; they become the body's signal of disequilibrium pushing into awareness, and providing the opportunity for exploration, expression or resolution. Understandably, many people are not able or willing to make this kind of reclamation as it involves feelings or conflict that are painful to acknowledge. Those who do so may only be able to make this transition with much support and guidance.

How a person experiences, conceives and communicates physical distress and how the helper intervenes may be represented as in the table, below. Generally, traditional medical disciplines and skills operate best at positions (1) and (2) on the spectrum. Here the concept of illness is dealt with as an alien or malevolent intrusion into the self. Position (4) is juxtaposed to these in regarding illness as an expressive syndrome. Position (3)— 'it's just your nerves'—is an interesting midway point; in return for the patient assuming partial responsibility for his dilemma, the doctor offers him a metaphorical structure upon which to hang this responsibility. A patient's 'nerves' imply an immutable and constitutional quality, and cannot be cured by the doctor as can an illness; nevertheless the patient may expect some kind of soothing or tranquillization of the metaphorical structure.

The psychosomatic-responsibility spectrum			
Somatic			Psychosomatic
Physical illness ①	Mental illness ②	'Nerves' ③	④ Reactive physical discomfort/disturbance
Responsibility Predominantly doctors		50% doctor, 50% patient	Predominantly patients
Psychological dynamic Encapsulation + internal projection to actual physical structure	Encapsulation + internal projection to assumed physical structure	Encapsulation + internal projection to metaphorical physical structure	Ownership and conscious conflict/distress
Language Physical structures	Psychological structures	'Nerves'	Distress described in ordinary language
Implied philosophy Determinism		Dualism	Monism/Holism
Nature of help Biological Engineering = 'doing to'		Support + social engineering	Empathy = 'Being with' + understanding experience working through
Intention of help Cure = destruction of illness via outside agency		Enhanced coping mechanisms 'learning to live with' disability	Growth = increased understanding. Resolving conflicts/relationship difficulties, thereby abandoning illness as an expressive and communicative mode
Perceived relationship to the 'self' External and attacking the self		Internal and compromising the self	Coexisting with and expressing the self

A clinical example

Let us take a simple and common clinical example to illustrate some of the features of this spectrum.

Mr A is a healthy young man who presents with cervical-occipital headaches for which no significant structural disease can be found. If he communicates his symptoms in wholly physical terms, and is accepted and dealt with at this level by the doctor, then both are functioning in position (1). The symptom is thought of as an excrescence; an autonomous disease focus to be cured or suppressed with drugs, while leaving Mr A himself immune from challenge or examination. The doctor calls Mr A's complaint 'fibrositis', and Mr A is pleased with this utterance as the mystifying nomenclature has taken his complaint away from him, and placed it in the province of medical science. The doctor has assumed responsibility for its definition and removal, and Mr A need not now worry about the meaning or nature of his bodily sensations.

Suppose, now, that the doctor expands his questioning and elicits that Mr A feels worried, wakes early in the morning, is sexually disinterested and often feels like weeping, but does not yield to this. He cannot, or will not, disclose to the doctor why this should be so and the doctor does not pursue the meaning for the patient of this disturbed behaviour or experience, as he feels that he has reached his diagnosis of 'depressive illness with somatic manifestations' (position (2)). The phenomenon is now encapsulated into a framework that implies a physical causation for the distress, though less tangibly or specifically than in position (1). However, the doctor's tone and language convey authority and a technical understanding of the patient's experience, which both lie beyond the patient's sphere of influence. The doctor, in treating 'depressive illness', has assumed the bulk of the responsibility for the distress. The patient's expected role is to remain cooperative, that is, to do what the doctor suggests.

Another doctor (or the same doctor on another day!) may not wish to assume this kind of responsibility. He may, too, be less convinced of the cogency of 'mental illness' as a workable diagnostic tool. He wants Mr A to assume responsibility for his plight, so he says 'Well Mr A, I've examined you and listened to your story and I'm quite sure that there's nothing seriously physically wrong with you to cause your headaches. I think we can put it down to your nerves. After all, you've always been a worrying type and you've also been under a lot of strain recently. Perhaps you need to take some time off work. These tablets might help, too, to relax your nerves'. There is an interesting shift in this consultation. At the beginning of the interview, doctor and patient conferred at position (1), but now the doctor has moved to position (3). He is willing to remain responsive to Mr A, but does not wish to assume total responsibility for his condition. If Mr A is responsive to this proposal, the consultation will move to a gratifying completion. Mr A will feel that he understands his complaint a little *better, and the doctor may feel that he has shared his clinical responsibility rather more, thereby reducing his own burden.*

But Mr A may not be amenable to such a move. He may deny he is a worrier, though his friends and family clearly experience him as such. Or he may say (angrily) 'Yes, I am a worrier but that's got nothing to do with these headaches, they're terrible, you know'(!) Assuming the doctor has been tactful and competent, Mr A's communication to him now implies something like 'I don't wish to explore the nature or meaning of my discomfort, and I don't want to take any responsibility for it'. If the doctor does not respect this defence, and persists in operating from position (3), it is likely that he and the patient will swiftly reach an unworkable impasse. The situation is akin to the child who does not want to eat what is offered; the feeding adult may 'know' correctly or mistakenly that it is 'good for' the child, but until the child himself is willing to take it, all attempts at feeding will be met by various forms of sabotage. Overt refusal, hiding the food in the cheek or napkin, or vomiting it back, all have their analogues in the medical consultation and the more complex task of psychotherapy. In the above example it is likely that the doctor will retreat back to position (1), confirming his act with a prescription as a token of his (albeit ambivalent) medical responsibility.

If Mr A responded readily to the doctor's suggestion of 'nerves', and showed an interest in how his complaint was associated with his feelings and relationships, the doctor may, if he has the time and interest, venture to position (4). If successful, Mr A will not be content merely to accept the label that he is a 'worrier' who suffers from 'bad nerves' but will want to integrate, understand and modify these mechanisms. He may see the doctor as a friend, a counsellor, a refuge in times of discomfort, but he does not expect technological magic or panaceas. In philosophical language he is perceiving himself 'monistically' and his distress as an expression of himself, for which he, ultimately has responsibility. Naturally, such a position can seem frightening and lonely; it is often far more comforting to experience oneself dualistically, and have someone else take care of our distress and difficult feelings, while denying that there is a deeper or more extensive problem.

It is interesting to observe how shifts in the spectrum may often work in the reverse way to these illustrations. In this case the patient will attempt to understand and integrate his illness holistically, while the doctor persists with a deterministic approach so that he can, without being undermined, assume his potent caretaking role (Zigmond, 1977, 1981, 1982).

I remember a previously healthy man, aged 80 years, who developed lobar pneumonia soon after his wife died; 'I think I got this because of the wife going', he said to the doctor, 'I feel so lost I just don't want to carry on'. 'That's nothing to do with it', retorted the doctor authoritatively, but not unkindly, 'your pneumonia is caused by the pneumococcus germ'. True, the old man needed antibiotics, but perhaps his diagnosis was also correct, and could have been advantageously pursued. In such instances it is likely that it is the doctor, not the patient, who is unable to integrate certain kinds of feeling; perhaps this doctor was uncomfortable about his own feelings of grief or loss.

In many medical consultations we are faced with this spectrum and options for changing our position. However, one of the rules of clinical communication is that consultation can only begin and go on with any viability if doctor and patient are operating from the same position and model. Likewise, there has to be accordance between patient and doctor for any shift to be beneficial; as the adage points out 'You can take a horse to the water, but you can't make him drink'. Reaching this common language and understanding is the central process in creating a therapeutic rapport. The route to such dialogue, as we have seen, is inevitably complicated by the distortions and resistances of both patient and doctor.

Mr A represented what Michael Balint (Balint, 1957) termed 'unorganized (non-structural) illness'. My next article explores how these principles may be applied to organized (structural) illness.

$$\Omega$$

Figures (1), (2) and (3) are modified from Bertrand Russell's *'Wisdom of The West'*. Rathhone 1959.

Note

The terms 'psychosomatic' and 'somatic' are used in a particular way in this text which may not be in accordance with other writers. Some literature implies that psychosomatic illness is 'caused by' the mind and its conflicts. This article uses the word in a different sense, so that mind and body may be seen as equivalents and not necessarily as cause and effect.

References

Balint, M. (1957) *The Doctor, His Patient and the Illness* Pitman, London

Bergson, H. (1911) *Creative Evolution*. Macmillan. London

Einstein, A. and Infield, L. (1938) *The Evolution of Physics* Cambridge University Press, Cambridge

Illich, I. (1976) *Limits of Medicine, Medical Nemesis; The Expropriation of Health* Penguin, London

Lowen, A. (1976) *Bioenergetics* Penguin, London

Perls, F. Hefferline, R., Goodman, P. (1951): *Gestalt Therapy* Julian Press, New York.

Russell, B. (1977) *An ABC of Relativity* Allen & Unwin, London

Russell, B. (1961) *A History of Western Philosophy* Allen & Unwin, London

Spinoza, B. de. (1955) *Ethics* Dover, New York

Zigmond, D. (1977): *Update,* 15, 675

Zigmond, D. (1977): *Update,* 15, 903

Zigmond, D. (1981): *Update,* 23, 1811

Zigmond, D. (1982): *Update,* 24, 281

Publ. In The Practitioner Vol. 226, April 1982

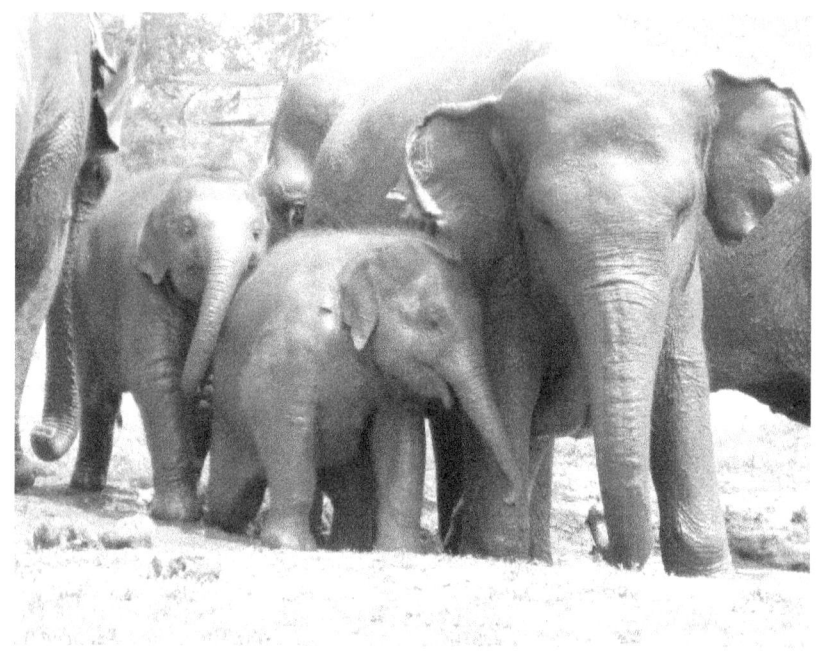

The Psychosomatic Mosaic

'It is the theory that determines what is observed.'

Albert Einstein

It is, perhaps, a universal wish to find, and relate to, an orderly universe, and yet the advancing edge of science always produces more that is questionable than answered. Medical theory and practice do not escape this principle. Whether it is cancer or the common cold, the mysteries of illness continue to outflank our organizing concepts. We find 'causational agents' – carcinogens or viruses – to explain disease and yet they remain partial explanations. Why does Mr H., who smoked only 15 cigarettes a day develop lung cancer, while his brother who smoked 40 remain clear? Why does Timothy develop a cold and not his four brothers and sisters? The traditional sciences, usually, have no substantial answers to such simple questions.

Levels of organizing concepts in illness

The quotation from Einstein is not just a philosophical principle. Our theories determine the configuration, content and outlook not only of scientific activities, but also our *personal* methods of experiencing and responding to the world. In medical practice this leads to professionally self-validating views and models of illness which are confined to the physical and deterministic. Analyses of illness are thus conventionally expressed in terms of anatomy, physiology, chemistry and the like.

There are, however, many other possible levels or approaches to illness, but they do not fit into this traditional mould.

Figure 1 illustrates how we may conceive illness from the level of subatomic physics to political theory.

Figure 1

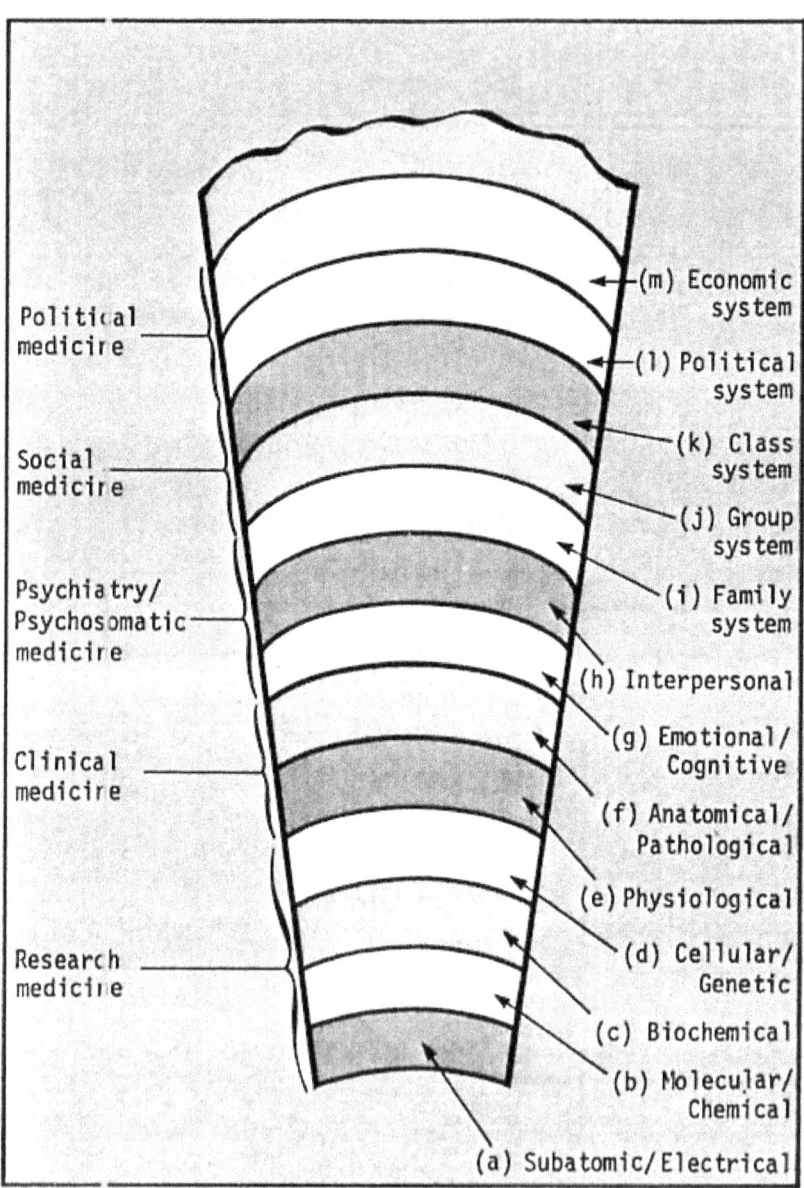

Levels of organizing concepts in illness

It is important to note that, although formulations at different levels may be dissimilar, they are not exclusive of one another; they are merely different levels, or angles, of observation and analysis. Much confusion has arisen because of our tendency to attempt to reduce our diagnostic and therapeutic formulations to only one, or a few, levels of organizing concepts.

Ascribing a man's duodenal ulcer to acid hypersecretion rather than his unresolved and repressed infantile hostility, may thus tell us more of a doctor's inclination, training and frame of reference than of the cause of the patient's illness. Our models derive as much from our psychology, as the world which we are attempting to define or influence.

Lord Kelvin, a once-eminent physicist, remarked 'If it works, it is true', and it is this pragmatic principle which should define the level and manner in which we operate in any particular clinical circumstance. Nevertheless, most doctors operate predominantly at levels (e) and (f), this being largely a reflection of the social definition of their role, and also how they see themselves; the image of potent biological engineer has its roots both in private fantasy and public expectation. Other levels of formulation and intervention thus tend, in practice, to be disregarded, avoided or dismissed, even though at times they may 'work'.

The reasons for such exclusion are both practical and complexly psychological. In practice, doctors often do not have the time, the expertise or the interest to pursue these other levels. Also the patient may neither expect nor want his doctor to perform anything beyond the traditional medical services. Yet deeper psychological issues define the pattern just as much. The doctor's fear of powerful feelings underlying the manifestations of illness, or his wish to exercise command over both his patient and what his patient brings him, are common examples. So, too, is the patient's wish to divorce his physical disturbance from its matrix of internal or relationship conflict; the man whose psoriasis gets worse when his wife goes on holiday alone, might be an example of this.

To illustrate how these principles may be employed in both diagnostic and therapeutic ways, a case history of a young asthmatic girl will be described. The letters in brackets correspond to the levels of organizing concepts in the figure. The ways in which the doctor might focus his attention and organizing concepts at different levels are also illustrated. Because of the author's interest, levels (g), (h), (i) and (j) are examined in greater detail. Levels (k), (l) and (m) are not considered to be in the scope of this article.

A 'simple' case of childhood asthma

Carol F, aged six years, was seen by her doctor at home because of her increasing wheeziness of one week's duration. This had become more severe, despite the competent use of antispasmodic, and later, antibiotic drugs. By the time of his visit Carol showed signs of marked bronchospasm and respiratory embarrassment ((e), (f)) and Mrs F was both agitated and anxious about her daughter's condition ((g)). Shortly before his home-visit, Dr V received a telephone call from Mr F. asking for a visit; the doctor felt Mr F.'s tone to be unduly threatening and accusatory, as if, somehow, Mr F blamed the doctor for Carol being ill. Dr V bore this with resigned stoicism and, by the time of his visit, had decided that Carol should be admitted to hospital, which he later arranged.

Carol had always been prone to chestiness; as an infant she had frequently been slightly wheezy and catarrhal, and Dr V had repeatedly treated this, with transient benefit, with the usual medicines ((c), (f)). He elicited the fact that Mr F's family had been prone to asthma, as had Mr F as a child, so he thought that Carol's complaint was partly genetic in origin (d). Dr V confirmed this hypothesis when Carol also developed flexural eczema, a sign of `atopic allergy', thus also showing a hypersensitivity component to her illness. Her increased wheeziness when the pollen-count was high in summer was another manifestation of this (d). In the winter, too, Carol would have more trouble with her breathing and *this was thought to be an allergic sequel to infections of her respiratory tract (d). Dr V had noticed how Carol was a 'very good' but quiet and introspective child (g) but he had explored this only so far as to say to Mrs F, 'Do you think Carol is worried about anything?'; to which Mrs F responded by turning to the little girl and asking rhetorically, 'I don't think so, dear. You're not worried, are you?'. Carol, duly hypnotized, nodded a whimsical 'No' to the avuncular Dr V, who asked no more.*

Dr V is a practical doctor who has little time to pursue modern thinking of prostaglandin activity or immunological aspects of the globulins in the role of asthma ((b), (c)). He is vaguely aware of the efforts of medical research workers in this area and recently was interested by an article which suggested that changes in the ionosphere could affect the electrical activity of cell membranes in vivo, thereby precipitating certain types of episodic illness (a). Dr V cannot make any use of these theories in his clinical work, though sometimes he wonders how these facts will be incorporated into future patterns of practice.

Dr V's observations about Carol's compliance and sensitivity were easily made. She is a slight, pale child who looks unduly timid and worried, and talks with submissive reticence. Indeed, in his dealings with her, Dr V had noticed how she rarely spoke for herself, even when perfectly able, her mother quickly interposing herself between Carol and the doctor, and then commandeering the dialogue (h). He thought this might be due, simply, to the effect of her recurrent illness and mother's ensuing anxiety.

Carol developed this attack of asthma, her worst ever, just as she was due to start at primary school; a fact which Carol and her mother were keenly aware of, but which had escaped the notice of Dr V. Had Dr V been attentive to this, he might have correctly supposed that Carol was 'anxious' about this important development in her life (g). And yet Carol's two other siblings, Brian (eight years) and Sue (nine years), never showed anxiety of this kind, so why should Carol?

Parental history

For many years Mrs F had seen Dr V for protean and ill-defined somatic complaints, which had little to suggest structural disease, but which he nevertheless, at first, investigated. Eventually he concluded that

Mrs F's complaints were 'functional' in nature. He experienced Mrs F as an anxious, taut and frightened woman, who seemed to radiate a sense of fear, urgency and wanting. In her visits to the doctor she would always refer these feelings back to her presenting physical complaints. On a few occasions Dr V had said something like, 'I can't find anything physically wrong with you. I think it must be your nerves. Is anything in particular upsetting you at the moment?'. At this suggestion she seemed uncomfortable, perhaps affronted, and with a blank look she would shift uneasily in her chair, foreclosing the interview by asking for 'a tonic' or repeat prescription.

Mr F, by contrast, rarely attended the surgery and, when he did, it was usually for a tangible medical complaint which the doctor could quickly and easily deal with. On several occasions, though, he had come with his wife, to amplify her complaint and underline her conviction that 'something must be wrong, and that Dr V must do something about it (h). At these times the doctor felt pressurized, and usually escaped from the corner into which he was being forced by arranging a hospital referral, which he knew to be unnecessary. Dr V is vaguely aware, therefore, that there may be important tensions in Carol's family which could be contributing to her illness. But within the context of his brief clinical encounters with them, he has been unable to define or use these patterns to either diagnostic or therapeutic advantage.

Let us look in greater detail at the members of Carol's family and the patterns that emerge at levels (g), (h) and (i).

Mrs F had always hoped for different things from her marriage. She herself is illegitimate, and was reared in a variety of institutions and by foster parents. So far as she knows, her own mother became pregnant at the age of 16 years, by an American sailor, at the end of the Second World War. The relationship lasted only a few months and, although the mother had wanted to keep her infant, her own wishes had been swept aside by the wave of her family's shock and indignation. As a child Mrs F was often treated kindly by her caretakers, but she was unable either to understand or predict what was happening to her, and developed a submissive wariness in her attachments.

By the time she was five years old she came to the conclusion that there must be something wrong with her, for her mother and father to have abandoned her. Failing to understand the complex reasons for the fragmented pattern of her care, it seemed to her that any satisfaction of her need for stability and love was sooner or later countered by unaccountable and sudden loss. At first she would openly show her anger and sadness over such losses, but eventually she thought it best to conceal her hurt, initially from other people, but later from her own conscious awareness.

As an adult Mrs F seems to cope 'normally' although, as we have seen, Dr V has noticed her hypochondriasis and tension. But to Mrs F, her life and relationships seem much more tenuous than an outside observer might suppose. Despite her apparent social integration, she describes her life as `like hanging on to the edge of a cliff'; in her dreams this is reflected by a 'terrible vision of falling into nothingness'. Her relationships are accompanied with much inner anxiety, in which Mrs F has a vague but ominous sense of imminent catastrophe. Socially, however, she seems merely to be rather tense and circumspect.

Mr F's childhood was very different, yet equally decisive. As the last (and probably accidental) birth in a family of eight children, he had a stable, but harsh, family experiences. By the time he was born, his mother was weary and his father resentful of the added responsibility brought about by his birth. It was not only food and money which were in short supply for the little boy but love, patience and attention. Mr F's father had a bullying and vitriolic streak and, by the time Mr F was a toddler, his father was using the boy as a vent for his frustrations. But Mr F was a resilient child and, rather than succumb to his father's dominance and sadism, he devised precocious strategies of avoidance and independence. As a schoolboy he looked to his friends for support and identification, and at the age of 15 years resolutely left his family for the Merchant Navy.

Some would consider it coincidence that Mrs F married a sailor. Psychoanalytic theory might postulate that she was trying to reclaim the father who had abandoned her. Transactional analytic theory would maintain that she did so to maintain a homeostatic system, where she could repeat the conditioned patterns of her childhood as this, paradoxically, represents security; the world she has experienced and knows how to handle. Whatever the explanatory theory, Mrs F is beset with the same feelings of insecurity and impotent wanting that she *experienced as a child. Mr F is a dutiful, though patriarchal, husband and father, a good provider and a source of reliable practical support when at home. But he avoids the finer nuances of trust and closeness, and Mrs F is mute in the face of her need for such emotional nourishment. As she confided once to an interviewing psychologist: `He's so good really, and he isn't often home; I couldn't really criticize him... I'd be afraid to rock the boat ...(!)'.*

When her children were infants, Mrs F found herself more serene, secure and satisfied than at any other period of her life. She felt a sense of attachment and belonging, which she wished could go on forever. For all their demands and inevitable episodes of difficult behaviour, her babies would continue to want her and love her as a mother. She sensed in herself a streak of resentment and sadness as her two older children became more independent and looked to other adults and children for their sense of belonging. Mrs F did not want to be abandoned with finality, and so Carol, as the youngest child, became special and precious for her mother; both a repository for her vulnerable feelings and a buffer against her own loneliness and fears of abandonment.

Although Carol had not yet the command of words or concepts to articulate her dilemma, she knew that mother was somehow frail and in need of protection. She sensed a danger in growing apart from mother, as if mother would collapse or stop loving her. Confronted by this wordless threat, Carol complied with what she sensed as her mother's demands. She became a rather clinging child, disinclined to contact with other children. When other children played in the street, Carol would rather keep her mother company indoors. Her physical illnesses could be seen as a somatic expression of her own, her mother's, and perhaps the whole family's conflicts. Her asthma both reinforced the bond between the child and her mother, and expressed the anger which she felt towards her mother for controlling and burdening her as she did. Carol often felt overwhelmed by what she experienced as her mother's needs, and sometimes in her fantasies, in an effort to be free, she would harm her mother or even make her disappear. Such strong images would usually bring in their wake intense feelings of fear and guilt because of what, in fantasy, she had brought about. Carol's asthma then seemed to her like a containment or punishment. In psychodynamic and interpersonal senses, her illnesses expressed and enacted the cycle of love, hate and reparation; her need to love and belong, her need to be separate and destroy, and her need to undo her destructive impulses.

Carol's illness has other significant functions within the family. It allows Carol to express the feelings of fear or helplessness for others, who can then disown such feelings in themselves and act in a responding and caretaking capacity. In this way Carol may be considered as a kind of siphon or amplifier for the unacknowledged, unspoken but important and persistent feelings of others.

Mrs F's covert emotional life has already been discussed, but what about Mr F? Perhaps Carol's illness might serve as a way for him to express both his tenderness and his frustration, which is so hard for him to share directly with his wife. Carol, as a constant focus of attention, creates a route by which Mr and Mrs F can both communicate and avoid one another; they talk a lot about Carol, but little about themselves. Carol thus becomes both a shared concern and a buffer between them. If they were deprived of Carol's sick-role, the difficulties between them would emerge more sharply and inescapably.

For Brian and Sue, too, Carol's illness has its functions. So long as mother's attachment needs are channelled into her care and concern for Carol, they are not discouraged from making other relationships outside the home and eventually growing apart from their mother. Should Carol become well, the mother's fear of separation would be transferred to them with greater intensity.

Table I summarizes a psychodynamic analysis of Carol's illness.

Carol	(1) Keeps mother loving and safe in the only way she knows how
	(2) Expresses anger and also reparation for her guilt from her fantasized anger
	(3) Makes mother and father seem closer together
Mrs F	(1) Keeps Carol close and special for her where Mr F has disappointed her
	(2) Helps her avoid issues of abandonment and aloneness
	(3) Allows Carol to express her own (Mrs F's) (unexpressed) vulnerability, fear and impotence
Mr F	(1) Allows him to show care and concern where this is difficult in other situations
	(2) Produces a common problem through which he can relate to Mrs F
Brian and Sue	(1) Deflects mother's oversolicitousness, thereby enabling them to be more autonomous
	(2) Makes mother and father seem closer together
The marital system	(1) Makes for a common bond between Mr and Mrs F when this would otherwise be lacking
	(2) Deflects feelings of neglect, resentment and uncertainty about marriage which would otherwise have to be encountered
The family system	Produces cohesion by:
	(1) Facilitating bond between Mr and Mrs F
	(2) Projecting otherwise disturbing difficulties and feelings into one family member thus leaving the others feeling unthreatened and unencumbered

Table 1:
Relational and psychological factors in the patient's illness

This table contains hypotheses which are inferential rather than directly observable, and this is generally true of psychological and psychodynamic formulations. How do we know if they might be true? There are two main methods which can be used.

Empirical and deductive method – Our hypothesis will make sense of otherwise disconnected facts, and predict usefully what might happen in future.

Deepening of rapport – Our interpretations, if skilfully conveyed to the patient, will lead to an increased thoughtfulness and increased disclosure and trust on the part of the patient in a manner which may bring about greater integration of split-off impulses and feelings, leading to change in symptomatology or behaviour. This will be examined further in the next section.

This empirical-deductive method of assessing psychological factors in illness is usefully illustrated in Carol's case. After hospitalization her asthma became much less severe, but she became seriously school-phobic and was referred to a child-psychiatrist, where the problem was eventually tackled in a family-therapy context. Her school phobia dissolved over a period of months, probably hastened by father's decision to change his job to that of a shore-bound ship's pilot. Although Carol's asthma became quiescent, and her school phobia resolved, her parents continued to attend the hospital for marital therapy, as problems were now emerging between them which they recognized as being theirs, not Carol's. This would be a likely prediction of the above formulation, and reinforces the notion of Carol's illness being the function, in part, of other family processes.

Level of rapport and the nature of diagnosis

If, as suggested, Carol's illnesses reflected unresolved conflicts and tensions at an intrapsychic and interpersonal level, how is an attending doctor to make use of this notion? As we saw, Dr V had noticed Carol's introspective submissiveness, the mother's overprotectiveness and hypochondriasis, and the father's rather truculent but protective attitude. He made a cursory attempt to understand the situation better by, for example, asking Carol `Are you worried about anything?', but this was met by mother's resistance in the form of denial. Perhaps the doctor's question was experienced by Carol and her mother as being too bold to yield candid exploration.

Psychological examination has intricacies similar to the physical examination and untimely questioning evokes a similar response to the sudden production of a doctor's cold hand on a frightened patient's abdomen. The doctor's shifting from a physical to a psychological frame of reference may have been too abrupt for the patient to adjust to and assimilate. It is now well established that response and compliance to taking prescribed drugs are significantly influenced by the size, shape and colour of the tablet or capsule. This principle is likely to be even more important in what we offer the patient verbally. How we offer an interpretation is perhaps more important than its content.

Dr V could, perhaps, have gone some way to bridging the gulf between his observations (Carol's passivity, Mother's anxiety) and the presenting complaint (Carol's asthma, Mother's hypochondriasis) by phrasing his question differently. With Mrs F, for example, he could say: 'I've listened to your story, and by examining you I can tell you that there is no serious disease causing your headaches. From experience we know that in many people the pain is due to tension in the body. With all of us, if we have strong or mixed-up feelings which we can't put into words or get rid of, then these feelings get stuck in different parts of our body, to cause tightness or pain. Sometimes I've thought that you look as though you have a lot of worry which you can't express or let out, so I wonder if you think this could apply to you?'

This form of question is more likely to be considered by Mrs F than the more direct, 'Are you worried about anything?', as it demonstrates the doctor's serious recognition of Mrs F's pain, and also offers her an explanatory link between her dualistic,* and his monistic,* frame of reference. If Mrs F were to pursue his suggestion, there follows a change in the level of rapport. Referring back to figure 1 we can see that her presenting complaint (headaches) is at level (f) – organ symptomatology – while the doctor's suggestion is at level (g), (h) or (i), depending on whether she chooses to focus on, for example, her own feelings (g), her anxieties about Carol (h) or the difficulties in the F family as a whole (i). If the level of rapport changes to one of the other levels, the diagnostic formulation will also change, as shown in table 2.

Level of rapport = level of organising concept of illness (see fig.)	Type of diagnostic formulation
(f) Organ pathology and symptomatology	'Functional headache' 'Atypical migraine'
(g) Emotional/cognitive	'Anxiety neurosis' 'Obsessional ruminations over loss etc'
(h) Interpersonal	Extended symbiotic attachment of mother and daughter
(i) Family system	Complex family tensions projected into somatic breakdown in two family members

Table 2: Level of rapport and type of diagnostic formulation

In the F family the level of rapport presented itself, and remained for some time, at level (f) so that Dr V. was dealing with Carol's asthma and eczema, and Mrs F's headaches, in a physical and dualistic manner, by conventional drug prescription. Communication between patient and doctor was confined to the events and language of organ disturbance and, consequently, diagnosis was in physical syndromes.

When Carol was first referred to the child psychiatrist because of her school phobia, she was initially seen individually and their communication was focused on Carol's fear of her angry feelings and the fantasies which she had of what would happen to mother, were she to leave her at home by going to school. The diagnosis now became that of the neurotic anxieties of the little girl.

The decision to take the F family into therapy changed the level of rapport again. The communicated problems led to a diagnosis of Carol's anxieties within a matrix of unexpressed marital tensions, whereby the mother's fear of Carol's separating from her reflected a displacement of the anger and hurt she felt towards her husband in this respect, and, reciprocally, Mr F's fear of closeness and the demands he felt which more substantial commitment would lead to.

All these observations and inferences are part of 'the psychosomatic mosaic'; no one part expresses the whole on its own and each part, ultimately, only makes sense with reference to its place among the others. Equally important, no one part 'causes' the rest of the picture to be formed, although it is true that at times one part of the mosaic will become more prominent and demand separate and complete attention. Carol's severe asthma attack needed immediate physical attention (level (f)) and an interpretation of her repressed anger (level (g)) at the time might be 'correct', but would certainly be untimely. Eventually, however, such an intervention made a substantial contribution to the holistic approach to her care.

The F family represent a fairly unusual example of illness in which the psychosomatic mosaic can be seen in a fairly whole form, albeit retrospectively, and after much professional time had been spent in broadening the rapport in a number of different contexts. More often the doctor is familiar only with one or a few pieces of the mosaic, perhaps because he is too busy and has neither the inclination nor the training to seek, or assemble, the other pieces. Usually such elaborate endeavour is not asked for, or needed, by the patient and would thus become an unnecessary professional burden or intrusion.

Sometimes, as illustrated by the case of Mr A in my article *A Psychosomatic Approach*, the doctor may wish to broaden the pattern of communication which the patient brings in somatic form, although the patient may steadfastly hold to his physical symptoms. Clinically we might label such a patient `hypochondriacal' or suffering from a 'depressive illness with somatic manifestations'. In psychodynamic terms the patient is employing a somatic defence whereby conflicts or impulses which are intolerable to the conscious mind or the patient's *modus vivendi* are split off and expressed by the body, leaving the conscious 'self' clear and unthreatened.

At times such a defence represents an acceptable and efficient working compromise between the self which is known, and the self which is forbidden. In these instances a doctor's zealous attempts to complete the mosaic would be fraught with difficulty; premature removal of defences is likely to be followed by a decompensation of the underlying psychopathology. Like inflammatory tissue, such defences are primarily protective and only secondarily pathogenic. A woman whose feeling of a lump in the throat, for example, is a defence against her unconscious wish to scream at and assault the dying mother she cares for, might be managed best along wholly physical lines; unmasking the conflict might be more than she can bear.

On the other hand, Carol F perhaps represented the opposite pole; the somatic defence was progressively decompensating and dangerous, but the underlying material was accessible and, with skilled help, could be worked through advantageously.

The question of when and how to expand our rapport and diagnostic image of patients is probably as important as the more traditional and familiar medical practices. The skills which we need, to be sensitive to such nuances, are as intricate, and at times as important, as any the doctor has learned in his conventional training.

*For the special sense in which the words 'dualistic' and 'monistic' are used the reader is referred to the previous article 'A Psychosomatic Approach'.

Publ. in *The Practitioner* Vol. 226, April 1982

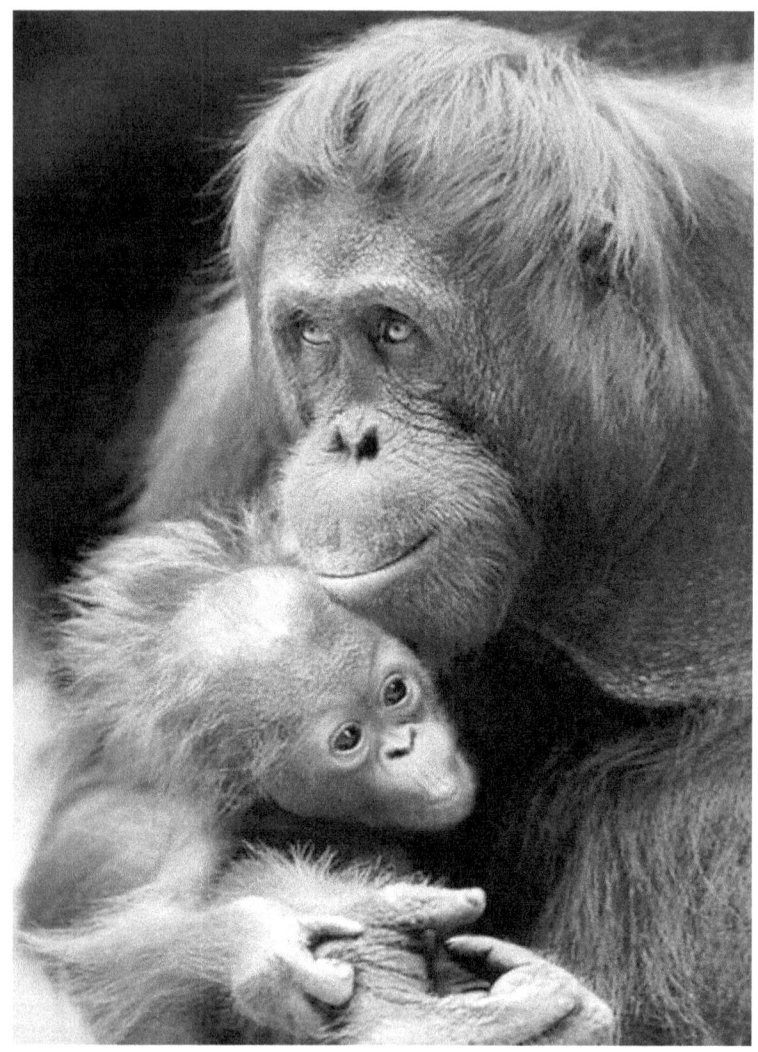

Mother, Magic or Medicine?

The psychology of the placebo

'Physicians must discover the weaknesses of the human mind, and even condescend to humour them, or they will never be called in to cure the infirmities of the body...'

Charles Caleb Colton, *Lacon* (1825)

It is not surprising that most contemporary observers and practitioners of medicine assume that drug treatment in medical and psychiatric practice is a kind of "pharmacological engineering". A sample of any text or medical dialogue concerned with this subject is likely to support the notion of the doctor in his role of engineer; his diagnosis locates or defines a malfunction in the body, and his medical treatment is applied as a specific chemical remedy. The practice that follows is guided by purely technical considerations— finding the most specific drug for the problem, working out its route, dose and timing. Explanations as to how drugs work are similarly inclined— replacing depleted chemicals, neutralizing acids, altering proliferation patterns in certain types of cell, inhibiting or catalyzing specific chemical interactions—are common concepts used.

And yet while doctors and medical researchers work painstakingly to refine such scientific theory and its application, the patients themselves often have quite a different way of experiencing the doctor and his medicines. For example, the evidence that most drugs prescribed outside a supervised hospital setting are not taken at all, or not as prescribed (Parkin *et al.*, 1976; Pearson, 1982) strongly implies that the doctor's "scientific" endeavours have quite a different meaning, or lack of meaning, for the patient. For all the technical talk amongst doctors of pharmacokinetics, serum concentrations, drug half-life and so on, if there is such a discrepancy between what a doctor assumes and intends and what a patient does, the questions arise "what is this activity, who is it for, and why does it exist?" For the doctor, prescribing in the prescribed manner has a number of functions. It helps him pass the time with the patient in a way that offers him the security of familiarity, and confers on him the mantle of "physician"; a cloak of potency, authority and legitimacy. It legitimatizes, too, his activities with his colleagues and gives him an identified place among them—they act in a similar way and so he is part of their group. It helps him feel helpful, even if this is not the help that is really needed; there are many studies suggesting this is often the case. The act of prescription may also provide the doctor with the comforting illusion that he is controlling or "managing" the patient's problem.

The foregoing indicates a little of why, for psychological reasons, the doctor may have his own compulsive need to prescribe. The main emphasis of this paper, however, deals with the complementary pattern—the psychology of the patient's need for drugs—which is equally fascinating and important. It is well established that placebos can have a positive therapeutic effect in a very wide range of disease processes in any bodily system (Doongaji et al., 1978). Placebo response to severe injury pain (Beecher, 1955) and angina (Benson and McCalle, 1979) are now classic studies. Severe mental disturbance in those labelled "chronic schizophrenic" often responds to placebos (Silverstone and Turner, 1974).

Some of the fragments of placebo psychology can be deduced from further research. A positive response depends upon an expectation of successful treatment (Lesse, 1962), a trusting and positive attitude to the administering doctors (Black, 1966), and the social status of the "healer" (Silverstone and Turner, 1974). In this latter study, patients with a demonstrated peptic ulcer responded symptomatically to a placebo given by a doctor (70%) but much less with a nurse (25%) The deeper and symbolic meaning of the placebo – which this article discusses later—has received less attention. Among the most interesting studies is that of Balint (1970) who studied, over a period of some years, repeat prescriptions in general practice. He concluded that the repeat prescription often represented less of a treatment than a diagnosis—that the patient was wanting protection and reassurance from the doctor, but not direct contact with him. Such patients were emotionally needy but afraid of a more direct or intimate contact, and so settled for this ritualized "dose of doctor" which represented a symbolic "something" that was "good, reliable, unchanging and always available". Clearly this need is similar, if not the same, to those needs of security and protection that run throughout our infancy and early childhood, and Balint here equated the drug's symbolic protection and goodness with mother, or earlier, the breast. Certainly Balint's notion was supported by the observation of protest, rage or crisis of some kind when the doctor attempted to stop or change the drug, usually with "clinically sound" reasons—the drug for the patient was not a mere "pharmacological agent", it was a symbol of caring, security and regard; its withdrawal seemed threatening to the patient, far beyond any possible medical implications.

Doctors' training generally does not involve recognition of these important principles, and certainly the skills by which they may be marshalled and used therapeutically have received little attention. The "rational", physical, components of prescribing have been pursued as a legitimate clinical study at the expense of those "irrational", psychological, determinants which, as we have seen, may be decisive, for better or worse. This indifference, or implicit contempt for the placebo, seems to have coincided with the "pharmaceutical explosion" in the 1950s (Doongaji *et al.*, 1978). It seems that the world of medical therapeutics reflected in miniature much wider social processes – a consuming and increasingly exclusive interest in technology, at the expense of psychological and social needs that have been with us since our beginnings. The consequences of over-investment in technology and attention only to the manifest, at the expense of more radical but hidden human needs, is an increasingly pervasive theme in our culture.

The following three cases go back to the "irrational" in treatment for their guiding principles. At first sight it might be easy to discuss them as in some sense "unscientific" or "quackery", but, on closer inspection, the skilful use of such situations and transactions involves some kind of applied science of the early mind.

Case No 1: A bridge over troubled waters

A 62-year-old woman, Mrs F, was knocked off her moped by a car emerging from a side-turning, driven by a young man, rapidly and without due observation. Mrs F was not seriously injured, but suffered painful bruising and lacerations. More troublesome for her were her symptoms of dizziness, shakiness, headaches and loss of confidence which the first doctor (Dr E) told her was "the shock coming out in you", and for which he prescribed a tranquillizer. A fortnight later she returned to see a second doctor (Dr G) saying she felt worse; she still had the same symptoms, but now she felt "unsteady and tired all the time". Dr G asked about the kind of thoughts and feelings she had toward the young driver, which led Mrs F to talk tentatively of her anger and resentment, which she had not previously expressed; "he was so kind and polite and apologetic . . . and I was too shocked at the time to say anything . . .".

But there was more to her resentment and sense of injury, which Dr G intuited from the little he knew of her. She had recently been made redundant from work, after 20 years with the same employers; they had themselves been "bought-out" by a younger and more aggressive company, which had decided to streamline the old order. At the same time, her husband had recently become ill with angina, following soon after his retirement. Her three children in recent years had married, moved away and become increasingly involved with their young families. In short, she was facing a period of rapid change and loss where the old order, and her familiar roles, were no longer viable or valued. Dr G had acknowledged and shared this dilemma with her, for brief periods, when she had seen him on two previous occasions. On this occasion, behind the miscellany of her physical complaints, Dr G was touched by the tears which kept welling up in Mrs F's eyes, only to be quickly dabbed away with self-disparaging apology. After an intimate pause of a few seconds the doctor said softly "I imagine your whole life at present is a bit like riding your moped. Trying to retain your balance and sense of direction while larger more powerful cars pass you by, often blindly, not aware of your vulnerability. It must have seemed like the last straw when that young man knocked you down. . . Perhaps it's unavoidable that you have strong feelings about this; if that's so, I think you'll need to face and talk about your feelings, rather than take tranquillizers to pretend they're not there."

Mrs F sat and cried for about a minute. Dr G was attentive but silent. This time she did not wipe away her tears, either literally or with apologies. "You've been a great help doctor, helping me express my feelings like that. You're right, they are my feelings and I do feel better just talking about them. I don't want a drug that 'gets into my system' —what about a good old-fashioned tonic?" Dr G's response, a prescription for a multivitamin syrup, was accompanied by his comment: "I think you will feel stronger and more able to cope with this. Come and see me next week."

Mrs F did indeed feel much better with her "tonic". "I know I have to get my confidence back myself, doctor, but that red medicine does me a power of good. I'd like it for just another week and then I think I'll be all right."

Her request complied with, her prediction proved correct.

Comment

What had Dr G done that was different from the first doctor, and can we deduce any scientific principles, even if in embryonic form, to account for his effectiveness?

Dr E had attempted to label and rapidly dispose of Mrs F's feelings by didactic reassurance and tranquillizers. He diagnosed "shock" without, in any way discovering what this shock had meant to her, and thus his verbal help could extend only to sympathy, not empathy. Dr G, however, had entered into her world a little, and understood something of her distress before making any attempt to change it. His intervention, when it came, was an empathic act; Mrs F felt validated and accompanied by Dr G in her hurt and despair. With Dr E, on the contrary, she had felt alone, alienated and discounted. Dr G had offered her, in a symbolic, brief but skilled form, an embracing and protective presence—those elements of successful parenting that all children need successfully, to pass through the many hurts and crises of childhood.

In the words of Guntrip (1964) "we do not grow out of childhood, we grow over it" and it is this Child within us that re-awakens and cries out in times of stress. Dr G sensed that it was not enough to give Mrs F adult reassurance, he had to somehow establish a dialogue with her inner Child, before the panic could be calmed. He knew also that her request for a "good old-fashioned tonic" was Mrs F's primitive need for a symbol of the doctor's concern, protection and understanding which she could take with her, and literally ingest, when he was no longer with her. Balint (1957) talked of patients taking "a dose of doctor" to describe the device of extending, symbolically, the therapeutic relationship. The following two cases explore this theme further.

Case No 2 A balm for grief

Mr D was 78 years old when his wife died. She had suffered a stroke two years previously, which had left her chairbound, dysphasic and dependent on her husband for all her domestic needs and the little contact she had with the outside world. Mr D provided this with great compassion, fortitude and humour, despite his own age and frailty. Her intense dependence on Mr D led to a strength of feeling and an intimacy between the two old people that had previously only existed

50 years before, at the beginning of their marriage. When she died, Mr D, despite his tears of grief, acted with the same courage and independence as before. Two weeks later, after he had completed all the funeral arrangements, he developed shingles on his chest wall and sought Dr E's advice. The doctor, after explaining the medical nature of the problem and offering a sympathetic warning to Mr D that he would probably experience several weeks of pain, sat back in his chair saying reflectively to Mr D "These must be hard times for you. I'm sorry I can't offer you more." The old man sat silently and sadly for a short while, looking at the floor. Raising his eyes to Dr E he said "I feel there's a big hole inside me—like somebody has taken something away." "Yes," the doctor concurred, "I think losing those we love does leave holes in us which we can never really fill in. Sometimes, though, with time, good new things can grow around the holes." Mr D smiled wistfully at his doctor before leaving with his prescription. "I think the talk with you is my best medicine, doctor. I don't feel so alone now."

Long after any specific medication could affect Mr D's shingles, he was continuing to want "something to rub into my skin" even though his skin was now clear and he had little in the way of residual pain. The doctor had at first resisted prescription, countering Mr D's request with a medical explanation of how it was impossible for a cream to now help his condition, which was largely resolved anyway. The old widower's eyes looked blankly at the doctor during his didactic effort, and then changed to an expression of hurt when he had finished. "I suppose you're right doctor but I feel ever so much better if I have something to rub in ... " Dr E now realized that it was not pharmacology that was required of him, but a kind of symbolic mothering. An inert cream, not recommended in any medical text, brought an expression of relief and seemingly inordinate gratitude from Mr D.

For three years the old man walked slowly round to see his doctor, to collect his prescription for his simple cream. He insisted on seeing the doctor personally; collection from the receptionist was not enough. The medical business of his consultations was perfunctory, the important transactions concerned the sharing, if only briefly, his world and feelings.

Mr D died alone, asleep in his bed, unexpectedly one night. Dr E was summoned by the neighbours to certify his death. Beside his bed were his dentures and spectacles, a glass of water, and a large pot of cream he had collected from his doctor two days earlier.

Comment

Mr D, like Mrs F, was facing a dramatic and painful change in his life. While more concretely-minded sceptics might claim that his outbreak of shingles was coincidental to his wife's death, it seems clear that the "treatment" Mr D wanted from his doctor was of some kind of representation of the doctor's understanding and permissive presence. Dr E had empathised with his aloneness and the grief and hurt that were expressed more by his body than by his words. The cream, for Mr D, was a way for him to have continuous, if symbolic, access to the palliative and nurturing presence of his doctor. The familiar religious symbols of Holy Bread and Water may confer on the believing recipient a sense of purification, forgiveness or strength; the clinical situation here is probably analogous, Mr D receiving from his cream a sense of caring attachment.

Many writers and researchers have stressed the importance of touch in the mental and physical development of the young child (Spitz, 1945; Harlow and Harlow, 1966) and the continuing health of the adult (Berne, 1961). Healing or palliative procedures based upon touch have a long history, and are still prevalent in Eastern medical practice. For the distressed infant, the touch of a protective adult is probably the most effective nonspecific remedy. Even as we grow older touch remains among the most potent and direct antidotes to pain, panic and distress. Mr D's choice of a "touching" medicine— "something to rub into my skin"—probably indicated a wish for this most basic of comforts, as a balm for the most basic of pains; the loss of a loved person.

Case No 3 Mother's milk

When Mr S, a solitary man of 40 years, became the centre of an angry cacophony in Dr T's waiting room, the doctor became apprehensive, but was not surprised. Mr S, he knew, had a lifelong tendency to violent outbursts, though never before with the doctor or his staff. Most previous contacts with the doctor had been for fairly simple requests, and on these occasions Mr S had had a rather submissive, faltering and lost manner; Dr T had the fleeting mental image of a small boy searching for a (his?) father. Dr T could recall other times when Mr S had come for "tonics" or hypnotics; the preceding events had usually followed a similar pattern: he would react impulsively and sometimes violently to a real or imagined slight or rejection, to be followed by a period of remorse, confusion and despair. Predictably, he was often unemployed, had spent several short periods in prison, and lived alone, as no partner could tolerate his periodic and explosive violent tantrums. After such episodes Mr S would seek help from his doctor, and would bring with him an air of injured dejection and deflation. It was at these times, in a rather piecemeal way, that Dr T learned something of the life of this hurting and hurt man. Mr S had suffered from the most elementary and early of hurts—the loss of both parents before he could remember. An accidental and illegitimate conception, he had spent his childhood from infancy in a variety of threadbare orphanages and, later, borstals. As far back as he could remember, he had been haunted by the fact of his early rejection, and had developed a primitive and only partially conscious notion of others as being untrustworthy and hurtful; a notion which he would spuriously validate for himself by provocation. Ten years previously, following a depressive reaction to one of his destructively cathartic episodes, a local psychiatrist had referred him to a unit specializing in a therapeutic community approach to "psychopaths". To Mr S's further sense of injury, he was rejected for having "insufficient insight or motivation to make use of the group-therapy approach."

The affray occurring in the waiting room at first involved only the receptionist. Dr T had no appointments left that morning except for "genuine medical emergencies", which did not seem to apply to Mr S, as the receptionist tried patiently to explain to him while offering an appointment that afternoon. The receptionist's positive efforts were rapidly swept away by a rage in Mr S that could not be reasoned with. "I DON'T CARE," he bellowed, "I'VE GOT TO SEE THE F_____ DOCTOR NOW." The doctor, his more routine and polite consultation quickly terminated, and realizing he was dealing with an emergency (even if not "genuinely medical"), entered the waiting room, much to the relief of his rather frightened and confused receptionist. "You seem to be very upset about something, and if you wait for only about half an hour I'll have some time for you . . ." While saying this the doctor looked directly at Mr S while putting a hand firmly but comfortingly on his shoulder; he felt Mr S instantly stiffen at his first touch, and then yield a second later, as if he suddenly found a sense of trust and acceptance in his doctor.

"I have this terrible feeling doctor, I'm afraid I'll explode, go mad and kill somebody . . . I'm afraid of what I may do . . . I didn't know who else to tell." The doctor, asking Mr S to describe recent events, established that he was reacting, again, to an event which Mr S interpreted as being a personal slight and rejection. It was, in reality, more likely to be the inflexible, but impersonal, bureaucracy of the Social Security Office. After talking for some minutes of the variety and threatening intensity of his feelings, Mr S sat back in his chair exhausted, lost and on the point of tears. Pausing deliberately, Dr T then said quietly: "You know, I imagine that all these feelings you have are the same ones you had when you were a little boy and you felt unloved and that something bad was going to happen to you. I think at those times life really did hurt you in a way you couldn't understand, and all those experiences have led you to thinking that the same kind of things are happening to you now, even when they're not ... and then you get all those old feelings crowding in on you. That desperate and unhappy little boy in you wakes up, and cries out, and starts fighting for his life . . ."

"That's true, that's exactly how I feel . .. But what can I do, doctor?" replied an attentive and thoughtful Mr S.

"Well, what would the 'grown-up you' want to say to the 'little boy you', knowing what he does?"

"I see what you mean ... I've never thought about it like that ... I think I'd like to say to him `You really had it rough and I feel sorry for you ... but you're the past and I mustn't let you run my life now' ... But how can I do that, doctor, I mean when I get upset I just see red and get mad and lose control of myself. I just can't help it ..." Mr S pleaded.

Dr T was insistent, if kindly, in his disagreement of this last statement. "Well, I don't agree that you can't control your actions. You can, but I understand that it's very hard for you and that you may need some help. I have an idea to help you, but it will only work if you want it to, and if you follow my instructions carefully. Will you do that?" he asked, looking at Mr S steadily.

"Yes, I will . .. I do want to try something. . ."

"What I suggest to you is simple but you must do it properly for it to work. When you feel the beginning of one of your strong feelings of panic or anger you must sit down quietly somewhere and suck one of the tablets I'm going to give you. Suck it and don't swallow it whole; you'll find it has a soothing effect as it goes down, first in your throat and then in your chest and stomach. When you're sitting there I want you to think about what we've been saying, and to have an imaginary talk with that little boy inside you. The tablet will calm you when you're doing this." At this point Dr T reached forward to touch the hand of Mr S briefly but significantly. "I'll give you 40 tablets to begin with and I want you to come and see me at the end of the week to let me know how you are."

Dr T's prescription was simple but thoughtfully chosen – a more uncommon antacid/antiflatulent tablet with a pleasant milky flavour.

Mr S two weeks later claimed that "those tablets have really done the trick. I know that if I've got them with me and do what you say then I won't get so upset or 'blank out' ... " He returned every few weeks to collect some more tablets and to talk with the doctor who would reinforce Mr S's new patterns and help him, in a piecemeal kind of way, with the thoughts and internal dialogues Mr S discovered, often while sucking. Two years later Dr T's unusual therapy had proved its underlying psychological theory. Mr S had not been radically transformed as a personality but he had sustained those important controls which enabled him to hold a single job for longer than at any previous time and remain free of the kind of violent outbursts that had been his previous hallmark. The price of this was a limited psychological dependence on his doctor and his antacid tablets.

Comment and Conclusion

There are a number of principles and metaphors we may use to describe and explain how this doctor made effective and sophisticated use of the most basic therapeutic tools.

He recognized that the disturbance in Mr S was occurring at an early child, even infantile, level of his mind, and that his communications had to be made accordingly. Reasoning, threatening or bargaining with Mr S's "grown up" part had been tried many times before and never with success. On the hypothesis that the outwardly aggressive Mr S harboured an inwardly frightened child reacting to some fantasized danger, Dr T knew that he must quickly make an alliance or rapport in a way that was both age and feeling appropriate. The careful choice of touch, simple words and eye- contact were designed to engender feelings of security and inclusion in Mr S, who was previously feeling alienated and turbulent.

It was not enough for Mr S to be "tranquillized" in this way only while receiving Dr T's attentions. His life had to be lived outside the consulting room, and Dr T had to find a way of helping his patient take with him an internalized representation of the doctor, which he would re-evoke at crucial times of stress and threat. Common notions of hypnotism usually call to mind formal procedures of trance-formation, but hypnotic suggestions may be made in ways far more various and subtle, as much recent work indicates (Brander and Grindler, 1975). Dr T's deliberate emphasis of certain words, pausing at certain times and touching Mr S when he wished to make a particular impact, were all ways of "anchoring" his message, of making a lasting hypnotic-association and imprint (Brandler and Grindler, 1979).

Long after the infant has drawn nourishment from his mother's breast, he continues to draw a sense of comfort and security from the use of his mouth, particularly when sucking. The persistence of this need into adulthood is often masked, channelled and ritualized, but remains ubiquitous. Dr T used this most natural of tranquillizers very directly in his choice of a white, sweet "sucking" medicine, and in doing so also took the opportunity to reinforce and anchor his earlier (hypnotic) suggestion.

As we grow into early childhood we have, increasingly, to learn to live without mother's omnipresence and undivided attention. This difficult process of separation is often accompanied by various manifestations of fear, protest and anger on the child's part, and he may often turn to an inanimate object as a source of solace. Teddy-bears, dummies, blankets are all familiar "transitional objects" (Winnicott, 1958), helping the child face the unknown outside world. The child confers on the object special powers that once belonged only to mother. This need, too, persists into adulthood and is likely to become more intense in periods of stress and loss, where those much earlier feelings of peril and aloneness are reawakened. All three cases described illustrate the process where the doctor's medicine had become a kind of transitional object. Mr D *(Case No 2)* faced his last years accompanied, not by a loved-one by his side, but by a tub of cream into which he projected loving qualities; a rather sad substitute, perhaps, but one which brought him great comfort.

In the film *The Wizard of Oz* the young heroine, Dorothy, believing in the Wizard's powers, finds resources and courage in herself with which to confront the Wicked Witch of the West. She does not know, at first, that the Wizard is only an ordinary man with no more power than she; it is her belief in him which enables her to face those things she would have previously fled from. These principles, too, lay behind the successful placebo-effect in all three cases, and are well substantiated by experimental evidence (Lesse, 1962; Black, 1966; Silverstone and Turner, 1974).

The last principle I wish to outline is quite as important in practice. In the cases described, the practitioners entered into their patients' mental world, in an intuitive and empathic manner, before confidently prescribing the placebo. Recent investigators (Balint and Norell, 1972) described what they termed 'The Flash' in the medical interview where the doctor, leaving behind the usual protocol and ritual, is freer to understand the inner and existential dilemma behind his patient's presenting complaints. While this often seems an essential component of successful placebo prescription so, too, is the skilled application of principles of how the child's mind develops (developmental psychology), and how this "child-residue" is manifest and operating in the adult (psychodynamics and psychopathology). This is particularly so when dealing with the kind of character problems illustrated by Mr S. The other two cases, depicting some kind of life crisis amidst periods of rapid change and loss, but against a background of otherwise stable personality structure, are undoubtedly easier to deal with but involve similar qualities of interest, flexibility, dexterity and genuineness from the practitioner. It is interesting to note that these seem to be the most important elements of effective psychotherapy generally (Truax *et al.*, 1966). Some practitioners might object that such endeavours are too time consuming to be practical. It is noteworthy, however, that even the relatively complex but crucial interview with Mr S took a little over 25 minutes. Dr T would probably have spent more time and energy dealing with the repercussions, had he refused to see his desperate but accessible patient.

Others might balk at the very idea of placebos, all too frequently used ineffectively and crudely as an act of blind, simplistic reassurance or, worse, a cynical and deceptive "quick trick" to get rid of a "troublesome" patient, under the guise of being helpful. However the intention and (lack of) scientific basis lying beneath such patterns of practice are quite different from the three cases described, where the process of diagnosis and selection was of quite a different order; they should not be confused.

In an age obsessed with increasingly complex technological activity and accompanying official (often vacuous) slogans such as "The Treatment of the Mentally Ill in the Community" it is often a valuable challenge to re-examine and develop those more intimate and human skills that, despite protean fashions in technology, remain a cornerstone of practice. Healing involves far more than physical engineering. The placebo effect serves well as an example.

$$\Omega$$

References

Balint, M. (1957) *The Doctor, his Patient and the Illness.* London: Pitman.
-- (1970) *Treatment or Diagnosis. A Study of Repeat Prescriptions in General Practice.* London: Tavistock.
--& Norrell, J. S. (eds., 1972) *Six Minutes for the Patient.* London: Tavistock Publications.
Bandler, R. & Grindler, J. (1975) *The Structure of Magic I & II.* Science & Behaviour Books.
-- (1979) *Frogs into Princes.* Utah: Real People Press.
Beecher, H. (1955) The powerful placebo. *Journal of the American Medical Association*, 159, 1602-1606.
Benson, H. & McCallie, D. P. Jr. (1979) Angina pectoris and the placebo effect. *New England Journal of Medicine,* 300, 1424-1429.
Berne, E. (1961) *Transactional Analysis in Psychotherapy.* New York: Grove Press.
Black, A. A. (1966) Factors predisposing to a placebo response in new patients with anxiety states. *British Journal of Psychiatry,* 112, 557-567.
Doongaji, D. R., Vahia, V. N., Bharucha, M. P. (1978) On placebo responses and placebo responders. A review of psychological, psycho-pharmacological and psychophysiological factors I & II. *Journal of the Postgraduate Medical Association,* 24, 91-97; 147-157.
Guntrip, H. (1964) *Healing the Sick Mind.* London: Allen & Unwin.
Harlow, H. F. & Harlow, M. K. (1966) Learning to love. *American Scientist,* 54, 244-272.
Lesse, S. (1962) Placebo reactions in psychotherapy. *Diseases of the Nervous System,* 23, 313-319.
Pearson, R. M. (1982) Who is taking their tablets? *British Medical Journal,* 285, 757-758.
Parkin, D. M., Henney, C. R., Quirk, J. & Crooks, J.
(1976) Deviation from prescribed drug treatment after discharge from hospital. *British Medical Journal,* 2, 686688.
Silverston, T. & Turner, P. (1974) *Drug Treatment in Psychiatry.* London: Routledge & Kegan Paul.
Spitz, R. (1945) Hospitalism. Genesis of psychiatric conditions in early childhood. *Psychoanalytic Study of the Child,* 1, 53-74.

Truax, C. B., Wargo, D. G., Frank, J. D. *et al.* (1966) Therapist empathy, genuineness and warmth and patient therapeutic outcome. *Journal of Consulting Psychology*, 22, 331-334.

Winnicott, D. W. (1958) *Collected Papers.* London: Tavistock Publications.

Publ. in *British Journal of Holistic Medicine*, December 1984

Physician Heal Thyself

The Paradox of the Wounded Healer

The 'caring professions' suffer from higher levels of psychological morbidity, suicide and marital breakdown than many other social groups. The reasons for these excesses are explored. A model taken from transactional analysis is used to describe the *malignant symbiosis* that may develop between doctor and patient as the result of the doctor's background, upbringing and medical training. Suggestions are made as to how the re-thinking of medical attitudes towards patients, but even more so towards doctors themselves, might help to prevent the syndrome of the 'wounded healer'. The integration of the 'masculine' and 'feminine' aspects of the doctor's make-up is essential in this regard.

'The stoical scheme of supplying our wants by lopping off our desires, is like cutting off our feet, when we want shoes.'

Jonathan Swift, *Thoughts on Various Subjects* (1711)

Those who care for others, out of vocation or compulsion, often have difficulties in caring for themselves. Doctors are notoriously 'bad' patients, and the doctor who is required to help a sick colleague is likely to be himself confused and distressed by the complex tangle of feelings and distorted communications that follow. In the last two decades there have been many interesting, though ominous, studies on the morbidity and troubles of doctors. Perhaps the most striking data concern suicide statistics. All the studies concur in demonstrating a rate of suicide among doctors that is at least double that of the rest of the population (Rose and Rostow, 1973; Editorial, 1974). It is significantly higher than comparable economic and 'non-helping' professional classes. Among hospital doctors, the highest rate is found amongst psychiatrists, followed by physicians, surgeons and, finally, paediatricians (Blackley *et al.*, 1968; Rich and Pitts, 1980). Studies from the USA imply that psychiatrists, overall, are more likely to commit suicide than their patients.

In concurrence with suicide, the rate of drug abuse and marital breakdown amongst doctors is similarly high (A'Brook *et al.*, 1967; Vincent *et al.*, 1969; Editorial, 1970; Vaillant *et al.*, 1970; Emschwiller, 1973). Quite as important, though less easy to measure, is the common tragedy of 'marital dry-rot'. By this I mean the marriage that has atrophied in terms of emotional closeness, intimacy, and enriched sharing. As with the dry-rotted timber, the outward form may remain, but the underlying strength and substance has eroded – collapse or crumbling is a matter of time. *McCall's Magazine*, with its own brand of journalistic prophylaxis, warned its readers in an article entitled' Never Marry a Doctor' that 'Physicians are poor husbands, poor fathers, absent companions, prima donnas and about as useless in bed as an electric blanket when the power is cut off'.

Other studies are equally illuminating in filling the pattern. Doctors are more likely to break down than others, but usually do so in ways that are private and socially obedient; the formal diagnoses describing the doctor's difficulties are expressed in terms of *neurotic depression* rather than *schizophrenia* or *personality disorder* (Duffy and Litin, 1964; Editorial, 1967; Murray, 1977). They are less likely to be convicted of crimes of violence, burglary and causing an affray. Clearly, even in illness and distress, the doctor's exemplary persona remains intact. Doctors' frequent but concealed alcoholism repeats this theme (Vaillant *et al.*, 1972). Typically the problems will be borne and hidden by his colleagues and family, but the wider community will be left in peace.

Humanising the data

What can we infer from such statistics? It seems that doctors, together with others in the caring professions, are relatively incapable of acknowledging or allowing themselves the frailties they may look after so assiduously in others. When it comes to a crisis in our own lives, there are many doctors who prefer to be seen dead (literally) than in any way compromised, dependent or weak. Our armour of assumed omniscience and omnipotence has taken years to develop and is hard to discard. Many of us have developed a compulsive persona of exemplary independence, strength and rationality which we are both ashamed of and afraid to relinquish. Regression is for patients, not doctors. Both the structure and nature of many medical transactions and rituals create the illusion, and then conserve, the doctor's executive and emotional power. The medical model itself, with its didactic style of defining health, normality, sanity, pathology and therapy, is clearly a major vehicle in this authoritarian circus (Zigmond, 1976; 1977).

Clearly, it is not only as individuals that we suffer and perpetuate this dilemma. We collude together to minimise, conceal or deny these problems. The ethos of the stiff-upper-lip and coping-at-all costs is learned (by imitation and taboo) early in our training. It is ubiquitous, and played extremely hard, particularly in hospitals. How many of us have allowed ourselves to be openly depressed and comforted by a colleague? We are much more likely to maintain a stoical and inscrutable front and urge others to do likewise – unless they are patients, of course.

From my own experience, and from what other doctors have told me in psychotherapy, workshops or friendships, I can only deduce that there is a tacit and severe conspiracy of silence regarding this painful area. Traditionally, and still prevalently, the lack of emotional rapport and support within the caring professions is paradoxical but gross. Our expectations of ourselves and others to remain strong and intact, whatever the conditions, are unyielding, and frequently far exceed the conduct required for humane and competent clinical practice. Default from this Spartan code is allowed only in ritualized and contained settings. Publicly and manically it surfaces in the beer-saturated mess party. With more secrecy and restraint – commonly if the doctor is a psychiatrist – it appears in the framework of psychotherapy which can, in any case, be claimed as 'part of his training'. However, in many ways what he is doing is stealing away to a special place where, in total privacy, someone will listen to, and accept, the vulnerable, dependent and sometimes violent parts of himself. He is paying someone to respond to him as a permissive and feeling person. It is remarkable and ironic how other groups who claim no expertise or particular concern about human suffering, such as ourselves, cope with it so much better in their own groups. The emotional support, accommodation and latitude that people allow one another in shops, industrial organisations and so forth, frequently outstrip our equivalent performance and attitudes within the caring professions. The following account illustrates the tragic nature of such collusive and defensive responses.

The case of Dr X

Dr X was a junior hospital psychiatrist who started his first post in this specialty at the same time as myself. He had only just arrived in this country from the Middle East, had no family or friends here, and was resident in the hospital. As a late recruit to medicine he was in his mid-thirties, despite his junior status. His manner at work was tense, obsessional, earnest and very introverted. He seemed an extremely lonely man, who spent his off-duty time either studying or impassively watching television in the Doctors' Mess.

Over the months he became increasingly capricious, prickly and withdrawn. Nursing staff became uneasy with his odd and irascible behaviour with patients. On one occasion he sprinkled a patient with water while chanting from the Koran, explaining to an attendant nurse that 'the patient's being would be made pure'. This was followed by his writing a long, untrue and defamatory account about another doctor in a patient's case notes. Largely to satisfy the nursing staff's insecurity, it was decided that Dr X's clinical responsibility should be undertaken by another doctor. However, this was done in an oblique manner, so that Dr X was not confronted directly with the concern that was felt about him, and he continued official tenure of his post. This strategy seemed designed to 'paper over the cracks' so that no one needed to encounter the alienated and unstable Dr X until his contract had expired.

At this point I asked to see Dr Y, the senior consultant at the hospital. Although inexperienced, I was clear in my view that this approach was not only confusing and jeopardising to patient care, but that Dr X's increasing paranoia and depression required more in the way of concern, compassion and confrontation. I said that, for fear of encountering him in this way, Dr X was being treated with duplicity, and this fed into his sense of mistrust, powerlessness and alienation. It would be far better, I suggested, openly to acknowledge his painful and serious difficulties, to relieve him of his work in a decisive and kindly-parental way, and find him help outside the hospital. Dr Y's response was authoritarian, defensive and dismissive. I was made to feel that such a breach of conspiracy of silence was inept, impudent and unethical. I was sent on my way. Dr X, soon after, died from a suicidal overdose while still an employee of the hospital. It is doubtful that this man would have died amidst these circumstances in any other than a 'caring' profession. He would have received help.

Doctors' dilemmas

Doctors in clinical practice are confronted by some of the most private, primitive and powerful experiences that can be shared with another. Consider the following perennial situations that many of us become seasoned to:

Mr A has cancer and he does not know. What should I say? Shall I tell him, or if not he, his wife?

Mrs B's condition warrants my exploring her vagina and rectum.

Mr D has had ulcerative colitis for 10 years. I think he should now have his colon removed and be left with a life-long ileostomy.

I will not resuscitate Mr E. The probable quality of his future existence seems unworthwhile to me.

I don't understand Mrs F's sexual problem. I shall ask her about her masturbatory fantasies.

Although Mrs G. denies any problem, does not want treatment and has committed no crime, I postulate a mental illness, which puts her at risk. I will have her taken to an institution and treated against her will.

Each of these cameos is dramatic or devastating for the patient, but paradoxically commonplace for the doctor. Being crucial and decisive for our patients, our licensed tools and protocols are correspondingly powerful and dangerous. In consequence we can only use them legitimately if we are, or at least seem to be:

- strong
- patient
- worldly
- sagacious
- unselfish
- responsible
- impressively knowledgeable
- highly ethical and scrupulous
- uncorrupted by power, aggression, sexuality and greed
- always intact and alert to the most demanding and diverse situations.

Conversely in the face of such demands we cannot be:

- demanding for ourselves when others need us
- unable to face what is there
- uncomprehending
- self-indulgent
- indecisive
- ignorant
- weak.

Such formidable requirements tend to involve 'blocking-out', or at least controlling to an extreme degree, natural feelings and actions that would otherwise emerge. Disgust, fear or overwhelming sadness may be spontaneous, healthy and authentic reactions to situations that are unsavoury, offensive or tragic. The doctor's armour of detachment and continence is necessary – at least in part – if he is to get on with the job. The desensitising effect in doctors by constant exposure to pain, distress, tragedy and horror has yet to be studied in depth, but I believe it frequently to lead to a kind of emotional anaesthesia or woodenness. It may be impossible to remain a vulnerable, feeling or spontaneous person when subject to years of these kinds of demands and controls. Perhaps doctors become hardened and petrified in the same way as professional soldiers. The effect it has on intimate relationships is then, predictable, for, above all, intimacy derives from spontaneity, emotional expressiveness and accessibility. It is not possible to be close to someone who is relentlessly sensible and responsible. They may seem more, but are really less, than human.

Transactional analysis; an organising language

I want here to divert briefly, and present in an extremely simplified form, the concept of 'ego-states' from transactional analysis, as my further points can be illustrated more succinctly using this language.

An ego-state is a system of thinking, feeling and behaving, all of which are interlinked. We all have three ego-states, although in each of us the content and strength of each ego-state will be different. The three ego-states are called *Parent*, *Adult* and *Child*. The content of the Child is largely complete by the time we are eight years old; Parent and Adult by adolescence.

The Parent develops from what we are *taught* by actual parents and other influential adults. It derives not only from what we are told explicitly, but also from what we observe them doing. The Parent is thus the seat of both *nurturing* and *controlling* impulses and behaviour, whether to ourselves or others. Subjectively our Parent feels protective or critical, and has the conviction of *knowing* what is correct and ethical, even when we might be mistaken. Generally, when we are in our Parent, we feel secure, and relate from a one-up position of 'right' and strength.

The Child, reciprocally, is the world of experiences and derivative thoughts and feelings that we had as children and re-experience and re-enact now. It has all the qualities of the unfettered natural child, as well as the child that has learned to adapt to survive amidst more powerful grown-ups. The Natural Child is fun-loving, pleasure-seeking, pain-hating, emotionally labile, demanding, impulsive, spontaneous, creative, curious, sexual, unashamed, greedy and loving. This part of us believes in magic, and may feel either omnipotent or completely helpless, just as we all did as small children. It is the part of us that shares and experiences with vividness and immediacy, and is thus the spring of our capacity for vitality and intimacy. As children, however, we had both to be socialised and to learn strategies of living with those we are dependent upon, and these dependent patterns of compliance or rebellion make up the Adapted Child. We relate here from a feeling of being 'one down', by justification, appeasement, rebellion or struggle.

The Adult is the reality principle in the personality. It is capable of observing, assessing, storing and patterning information in an objective way. It can turn these logical powers externally to the outside world, or internally to monitor and mediate between the other two ego-states. In many ways the Adult may be seen to function like a computer. For simplicity we can represent these personality functions diagrammatically (Figure la).

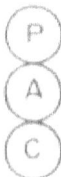

FIG. 1a—The three ego states. P = Parent—controlling, critical, nurturing, "one-up". A = Adult—Problem solving, logical, objective. C = Child—spontaneous, feeling, needy, creative, vulnerable, adapting to others, "one-down".

The doctor's personality

In the preceding sections I have reviewed both how doctors take better care of others' needs than their own, and how the nature of their work calls on them to be uncompromisingly 'grown-up' in their conduct. Using the ego-state model it seems that doctors' personality structure and function is confined largely to the Parent and Adult. We may spend our lives looking after those who are sick or compromised, and consider ourselves expert in knowing what is 'good for' others. Many of us pride ourselves on our accurate observation, fund of factual knowledge and problem-solving ability. What we are often out of touch with is our Child. The world of chaos, irrationality, strong feelings, spontaneity and vulnerability is kept strongly in check, if not denied and defended against, by our Parent and Adult ego systems. Such armour may at first serve as a protection, but such security is bought at the price of inaccessibility and shutting out the joy and intimacy that keeps us vital. A diagram of this process is illustrated in Figure 1b.

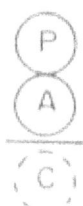

FIG. 1b—The doctor's personality. Strong Parent and Adult but blocked or atrophied Child.

Symbiosis – helping the needy and needing the helpless

When we deny powerful needs or impulses in ourselves, we will either be intolerant or compulsively solicitous of these attributes in others. If it is the latter, then we can professionalize this problem by working in one of the caring professions. In this area we have licence to seek out and look after the part in other people that we disown or suppress in ourselves. Our needs may then be fulfilled, in an illusory and vicarious way, through a state of mutual dependence. Such an interlocked relationship may be diagrammed as in Figure 2, and may be termed 'symbiotic'. Symbiosis may be thought of as 'benign' when our own needs are peripheral to 'helping the needy'. Conversely, 'malignant' symbiosis is enacted when our own needs become more central, and we are then 'needing the helpless'.

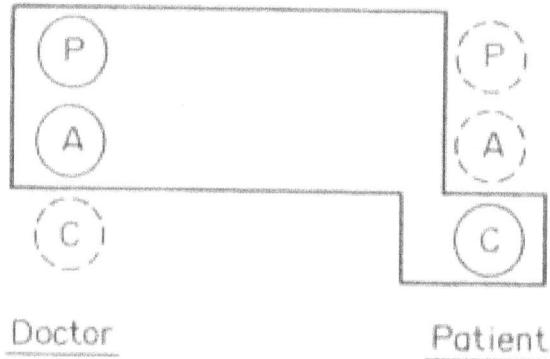

Doctor   Patient

FIG. 2—Symbiosis in the doctor–patient relationship.

There is a tacit contract here, where the doctor's part reads:

- 'I will be strong if you will be weak.
- I will be sane/sober/logical/continent if you will be mad/drunk/confused/miscreant.
- I will support, guide and protect you so long as you are helpless and obedient.
- I will not express my feelings or difficulties, so you must have and enact them for me'.

Reciprocally, the patient's role in such a collusion reads:

'If you will be my Grown-up then I will make you feel potent, clever and important (or, not infrequently, the opposite). To make sure that is so, I will be passive, aimless and dependent'.

Such dependence upon our patients for our sense of power, self-esteem, worthiness and vicarious expression of locked-up feeling is often not conscious. In the semi-conscious or deeply unconscious mind there are frequently complexes of guilt, and the need for reparation, stemming from our earliest experiences where, in a primitive and irrational manner, we created inordinate notions of the damage we might have done or might still do. Compulsive and malignantly symbiotic patterns of help then represent a ritualistic undoing of the feared damage, but it is an impotent undoing which is never finished and must be repeated endlessly. In the short term this kind of 'helpfulness' may be harmless. The long-term effects, however, may be similar to many other relationships which are based upon rigidity and a radically unequal power distribution. Because attachment and gratification of both partners depends on a rigid status quo where no growth is possible, a sense of entrapment, waste and resentment is likely to evolve. In the interim, it may account for many harried, irritated and depressed doctors who are uncomprehendingly or unconsciously dependent on their patients' dependence. The end point of this process is the unnecessarily infantilised or institutionalised patient and the seriously damaged, or prematurely dead, doctor.

The making and breaking of doctors

The factors that motivate us to become doctors are often those which later lead to the kind of stoical and compulsive unhappiness I have outlined. In this section I shall discuss briefly the kind of family and social backgrounds that make a radical and pervasive contribution to these difficulties.

Altruism, caring and empathic concern for others in distress are clearly ingredients of the most humane and proficient practice, and involve only benign symbiotic attachments, which is a necessary, if temporary, arrangement while dealing with distress and disability. It is the malignant symbiotic patterns that stem from the doctor's personal difficulties and lead, via his defences of workaholism, perfectionism and stoicism, to the even greater difficulties I have reviewed. In a general sense such doctors are likely to have grown up with the notion that it is forbidden, disadvantageous or damaging for them to express their feelings, make demands or be vulnerable, although they may be permissible or even expected in others. The reasons for this can, of course, vary from implicit social class mores to particular family circumstances. As an example of the latter, the following case history serves as an example:

The case of George

George is a physician in his mid-forties. He sought help originally when things were clearly going wrong in his life. In spite of his outward success, good professional standing and apparently stable family life, he experiences his existence in terms of deadness, hollowness, edginess, joylessness and inauthenticity. Clinically his problems might be described in terms of 'anxiety', 'depression' and an underlying 'obsessive-compulsive personality'. In more ordinary terms he is a man who works inordinately hard, is never satisfied with the work he has done, fears (unrealistically) any criticism from his colleagues or patients, and finds it almost impossible to assert himself or differentiate himself from others' expectations and wishes. His way of relating is thus usually either appeasing or reparative, but in being so, he accumulates much in the way of resentment with others (for their dominance), self-hatred and poor self-esteem (for his acquiescence) and alienation (from his inauthenticity). These consequences are expressed at home, where he becomes depressed, irritable and demanding, and periodically explosive with anger. His attempt to escape his passive-aggressive cycles via alcohol merely amplifies his problems of guilt, remorse, liability and despairing confusion. The effect on his marriage is seriously damaging and needs no further elaboration here.

George was born shortly before the outbreak of the Second World War. It is possible that his parents were never really happy together. Soon after his birth, his father was conscripted into the forces and saw little of his wife or son in the next six years. Even after the war the pattern continued in a similar way, as father was often away from home travelling in his work. George's mother was an unhappy and lonely woman who sought from her little boy not just the love expected from a son, but also the unavailable love she craved from an absent or unloving husband. During her lonely war years she took the boy into her bed, and when he was old enough to 'understand' she confided in him about her unhappiness with father.

By the time he was six years old, George had formed the decision that mother's stability, love and happiness depended upon his ministering to her. Family triangulations and oedipal conflicts are difficult to resolve even in less exceptional circumstances, but for George there was the added misery of inexorable and increasing alienation from father. Hardly surprisingly, father experienced the intense bond between his wife and son as an alliance against him, and indeed it was true that the closeness of these two depended on keeping father 'bad' or distant. The dilemma of the little boy was that he had to suppress his own feelings and needs and subsume these to another's, but that in doing so he necessarily drove father away or invoked his hostility. 'I just couldn't do the right thing; I couldn't make them happy' George recalls tearfully some forty years later, and it was certainly true that the task this little boy saw for himself was quite beyond his resources or understanding, or powers of influence. And yet he felt responsible and had to keep trying to find a solution.

He cannot remember now when he decided to become a doctor, but he does remember some of the thoughts that went with the decision. He would imbue himself with the powers of healing, but, in so doing, people would be genuinely grateful and thankful. Unlike his family (where he felt compelled to 'heal' his mother but felt bound to fail and instead collect feelings of guilt, fear and inadequacy) as a grown-up healer – a doctor – he would be potent, respected and unassailable.

Little George's compensatory and reparative fantasy has had very different consequences in grown-up reality. Not only did he not make mother and father happy or loving but, inevitably, some of his patients didn't get better. Often they seemed ungrateful, and occasionally they blamed him even when he knew it wasn't his fault. He responded with the same mixture of guilt, resentment and fear he had as a young boy, and tried harder. The characters and backcloth changed, but the theme has remained the same. George's malignant symbiosis with his patients can be seen as his attempt to solve archaic, and probably insoluble, problems within his family, but also, by identification with his patients, to get for himself the love, care and acceptance that were lacking for him. He compulsively gives to others what he has yearned for himself. In the long term, however, this route becomes a cul-de-sac, offering no real satisfaction or resolution. George's symptoms have signalled as much, and it has only been since he has been tackling and expressing his needs, wants and hurts more directly, and for himself, that he has begun to leave them behind. He has realised that charity must begin at home.

George's difficulties and their origins are, in my experience, fairly typical of the common syndrome of the *Wounded Healer*. Others have remarked on how doctors and psychotherapists tended to have had significantly depressed mothers eg Storr, 1979) which led them not only to an empathic understanding of this in others, but also, less helpfully, to a compulsive need to sacrifice the self in 'helping'. Apart from the current of guilt that underlies this impasse, there are other components of this syndrome which damage and distort our self-esteem. In seeing our lives in terms of what we offer to others, often in a very confined and ritualistic form, we do not value ourselves for what we really are, but only what we *do*. Such a central dissatisfaction with ourselves may account for much of our motivation in seeking out the compromised parts of others. In this symbolic union, we imagine, we can allay our own loneliness and sense of incompleteness. The cruel and inescapable truth, however, is more often the reverse. It is only through loving ourselves that we can enact creatively an authentic and discriminating love of others.

We need also to consider the way in which our social and class backgrounds contribute to these patterns. Doctors have traditionally been recruited from the middle and upper classes, particularly those which have a strong parental ethic. There is a tendency for this section of society to pride itself on knowing best what is 'good for' other members of society. We take the *Times, Telegraph* or *Guardian;* our experience of the world (and often the world itself) is for organisation, edification and improvement – not enjoyment. It is not only doctors, of course, who emerge from this patriarchal mould. We produce a plethora of other parental types: lawyers, clergy, captains of industry and politicians. We are prepared early for these tasks. How many of us can remember being told prematurely to 'grow up', 'don't be silly' or 'to be more responsible' when we were not yet eight years old, and childhood with all its tumult and selfishness should have been our right? Later, this false and precocious acceleration into adulthood may have been compounded even further by education in public schools, with its essential ingredients of rules, responsibilities, hierarchies and titles. In such environments, our emotional life or private world is regarded as a hindrance or aberration, deflecting or subtracting from our more important public performance. We thus become more oriented to achievement than experience; what we *are* is important only in so far as it is expressed in what we *do*. The 'masculine' nature of such cultures has a particularly inhibiting effect on the feeling, vulnerable 'feminine' side of ourselves.

I remember at the age of eleven standing alone with my 'tuck-box' on the station platform, awaiting the steam train to take me to boarding school. I was fighting back the fear and the tears, and trying bravely to look grown-up. Like George, I developed this concealment over the years, to become a 'false self'. Ultimately, it has needed dismantling before I could excavate and pay attention to the buried Child within me. Here, too, charity has had to begin at home.

Physician heal thyself – but how?

Official recognition of the disturbed doctor who may be a liability to his patient represents only a surface layer of a problem which, as I have outlined, is extensive and complex. Public concern about this problem has led, in recent years, to the implementation of the 'three wise men' whose task it was to assess, caution, make recommendations to, and sometimes discipline, the aberrant doctor. However, such a 'casualty department' approach, even if doing a little to protect the public, has little impact on the underlying and seemingly ubiquitous difficulties: these have their roots in deep-seated emotional problems and social mores.

The teaching of psychiatry via a medical-model didactic type of approach is now a well-established discipline conveyed to medical students. More recent, and less developed, is the introduction of the teaching of the psychology of the patient or the person who is ill. What is lacking in both of these approaches is any significant consideration of the doctor and his psychology and distress patterns. It is somehow assumed that these problems do not exist, or are insufficiently important to merit teaching time and expertise, or that somehow the doctor will muddle through successfully. Clearly, the facts indicate otherwise.

All creative acts can be interpreted in terms of some kind of psychopathology. Compensation, identification, projection, denial, escape and sublimation are some of the technical words we might use to describe the mechanisms lying behind many endeavours. The fact that a young person is prepared to spend many arduous years training to license himself for the lifelong task of involving himself with unknown persons' distress is, on the surface, a perverse choice and likely to be based, at least in part, on such covert forces. Yet it would be wrong to assume that these kinds of motivations need necessarily be problematic or pathological in practice. Very real gifts and predispositions for caring and empathy may arise from such factors in ourselves. Indeed, it is probably not possible to develop a humane and compassionate resonance with another unless we have some identification with them. We have to have faced similar pains, losses, conflicts or needs ourselves. The important point is that we are both aware, and in control, of these forces within us. By doing so we convert a liability into a gift.

Yet the medical educational establishments whose task it should be to help the medical student or young doctor successfully navigate these dilemmas and transitions fails to realise either the presence or significance of this task. By concentrating solely on the 'masculine', scientific, organisational and didactic aspects of the doctor's role, medical education falls short of being an 'education' and remains a 'training' – a constriction or moulding into the required role. What is lacking in this process is the more 'feminine', nurturing approach, where experience is accepted and understood at a more feeling level. It is only via this more candid and allowing attitude that the developing doctor will find himself in an environment where he can successfully engage and transcend what will otherwise become a series of impasses which become translated into the kinds of stoical, insensitive or malignantly symbiotic patterns of lifestyle and practice we have considered.

There are practical ways of achieving this. From the first day at the dissection table, medical teachers should consider it part of their task to encourage students to talk about their attitudes, feelings and problems. Clinical teachers should share with their students the difficulties they encounter in, for example, caring for the incurable, the inexorably dependent and the dying, or making mistakes! They might enlighten the students too, in discussing with them the human resources they have had to develop to deal creatively with these situations. Integrated into the curriculum, alongside the more formal and traditional teaching, there should be seminars or discussion groups where personal disclosure and interaction about these issues would be skilfully and sensitively encouraged. Many clinical teachers might, at first, be threatened by this requirement that they become humanistic as well as technical teachers. They might feel that self-disclosure would be undermining and would diminish their position of respect and authority. My own experience has been opposite to this. The teacher who can share his difficulties and humanity while remaining a master of his craft grows in the esteem of others and serves as a model as to how these things may be reconciled.

It is clear that many young and established doctors have needed, and will continue to need, professional help for the problems that are likely to emerge within them in the course of their careers. As I have demonstrated, this is to be expected as a natural consequence, at least sometimes, of the nature of ourselves and our work. It should carry no more stigma or alarm than the football player who needs physiotherapy to relieve his pain and heal him so he may again be competent for his task.

I have not said anything about the kind of social mores and public expectations of doctors, which feed into how the doctor feels he should be and compound his individual difficulties. This would require a separate article of equal length. However, I would anyway urge us to desist from this large and formidable task of analysis and intervention until we have our own house in order. We are, of course, already proudly 'expert' in defining what is wrong with others and what they should do.

Charity begins at home; physician heal thyself.

Ω

References

A'Brook, M.F. Hailstone, J. D. & McLaughlin, E. J. (1967) Psychiatric illness in the medical profession. *British Journal of Psychiatry,* 113, 1013-1023.

Blackley, P.H., Disher, W. & Rodmer, G. (1968) Suicide by physicians. *Bulletin of Suicidology,* 1-18.

Duffy, J.C. & Litin, E.M. (1964) Psychiatric morbidity of physicians. *Journal of the American Medical Association,* 189, 989-992.

Editorial (1967) Emotional illness in physicians. *Medical Tribune* (March 29), 1.

— (1970) Drug abuse. Growing occupational hazard for doctors. *Hospital Physician,* 6, 60.

— (1974) Suicide among physicians. *Journal of the American Medical Association,* 228, 1149-1150.

Emschwiller, J. (1973) Doctors still drink too much and pop too many pills. *Medical Times,* 101, 58-61.

Murray, R.M. (1976) Characteristics and prognosis of alcoholic doctors. *British Medical Journal,* 2, 1537-1539. [Not referenced in the article]

— (1977) Psychiatric illness in male doctors and controls: an analysis of Scottish hospitals in-patient data. *British Journal of Psychiatry,* 131, 1-10.

Rich, C.L. & Pitts, F.N. Jr. (1980) Suicide by psychiatrists: a study of the medical specialists among 18,730 consecutive deaths during a five year period 1967-72. *Journal of Clinical Psychiatry,* 41, 261-263.

Rose, K.D. & Rostow, I. (1973) Physicians who kill themselves. *Archives of General Psychiatry,* 29, 800-805.

Storr, A. (1979) *The Art of Psychotherapy.* London: Heinemann.

Valliant, G.E., Brighton, J.R. & McCarthur, C. (1970) Physicians' use of mood-altering drugs. *New England Journal of Medicine,* 283, 365-370.

Valliant, G.E., SobowallL, N.C. & McArthur, C. (1972) Some psychological vulnerabilities of physicians. *New England Journal of Medicine,* 287, 372-375.

Vincent, M.O., Robinson, E.A. & Lave, L. (1969) Physicians as patients. *Canadian Medical Association Journal,* 100, 403-412.

Zigmond, D. (1976) The medical model, its limitations and alternatives. *Hospital Update* (August), 424-427.

— (1977) Scientific psychiatry: progress or regress? *Update* (October), 675-679.

British Journal for Holistic Medicine, Dec 1984

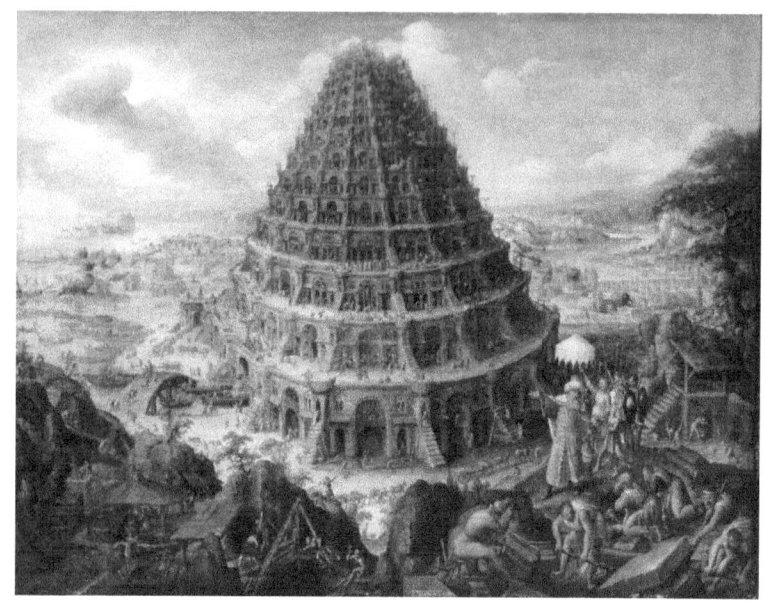

Master van Valckenborg the Elder – *The Tower of Babel* 1595

Babel or Bible?

Order, Chaos and Creativity
in Psychotherapy

'The quest for certainty blocks the search for meaning.
Uncertainty is the very condition to impel Man to unfold his powers.'

Erich Fromm, *Man for Himself*, 1947

Several years ago, an intelligent and troubled friend of mine – I shall call her Carol – then in her mid-twenties, was sent to a psychiatrist because of worsening symptoms of depression. She remembers him as a kind, fatherly man who asked her a comprehensive range of questions to survey her symptoms, life and dilemmas. Before she left, he informed her of his view that her pattern of distress would be 'best treated by psychotherapy', and that he would make arrangements accordingly. Carol, although a bright and educated young woman, came from a background largely alien to matters psychological and introspective. Her parents, pragmatic Northerners from an industrial city, represented a culture and way of thinking very different from the psychodynamically sophisticated psychiatrist she encountered; she did not know what psychotherapy was and he, perhaps unwittingly, did not explore this gulf between them. It was several weeks before Carol received a standardised letter from the hospital, telling her of an appointment with Dr L, a psychotherapist, in four months' time.

By the time Carol went to see Dr L her most troublesome depressive symptoms had largely subsided, perhaps due to medication she had been prescribed. She was, however, left with a churning, ineffable dis-ease inside her, which became heightened on the day of her appointment; the fantasy of her imminent meeting with Dr L produced an added, tense composite of hope and fear. A long period of waiting in a neon lit and threadbare waiting area preceded the appearance of Dr L 'Miss Jackson? I am Doctor L. Will you follow me please', was Dr L's sparse greeting. His voice seemed uncompromisingly dry and neutral, Carol thought, as she was led along a corridor and into a small, bare room in which there were two easy chairs. Dr L closed the door behind them and silently gestured to one of the chairs, as he sat down himself. A period of silence followed which, for Carol, was unexpected and increasingly uneasy. Her previous encounters with her own doctor and the psychiatrist had been in some ways embarrassing and difficult, but reassuringly structured by the initiative they took in asking questions, and offering explanations and suggestions of various kinds; at those times she had felt encouraged by the elementary support and interest shown to her. Dr L, however, seemed quite different – with the silence growing laden and unnatural, Dr L's gaze felt paralysing to Carol, and, when he turned his eyes to the floor, she felt unaccountably abandoned and unsafe. She had wanted to ask him what she was expected to say or do, but became increasingly anxious that she might be breaking some kind of unspoken code by doing so, although part of her was aware of the irrationality of the notion, Dr L's silence and inaccessibility in the face of her mute need and fear, had turned him, in her mind's eye, into some kind of omniscient and unappeasable giant that she could not now approach directly.

Perhaps ten or fifteen minutes passed in this kind of ominous wilderness before Dr L, shifting slightly in his chair, spoke with dry rhetoric: 'I suppose you're rather angry, but don't know how to express it'. 'Angry, why should I be angry? I just feel rather confused ...' pleaded Carol, disoriented and frustrated, imagining that she had somehow missed her cue, that he demanded some kind of 'correct' response that she had not been able to fathom or, therefore, provide. 'Confusion can be an excellent way of avoiding strong feelings when they seem threatening', came Dr L's reply, authoritative and consummate. 'But I still don't know what you mean. Who am I angry with?' replied Carol, beginning to find some kind of clarity and confidence, perhaps because this silent and inscrutable man was now, at least, speaking to her. 'Perhaps with the hospital who kept you waiting for an appointment so long. And then, again, with me for keeping you outside (in the waiting area) – isn't that what happened in your family, that they kept you "waiting outside", when you were sent to boarding school?'

Carol was slightly taken aback by his knowledge of her; again her fantasies turned to his omniscience, and her sense of his having a secret cache of understanding about her, and a hidden agenda with her, to which she was denied access. Bewildered by these potent images, she retreated to the more tangible suggestion that he made: 'But I understand the NHS system; I know that there are waiting lists for all kinds of services, and that I can't blame anyone for that. Anyway, I have been feeling rather better lately…', said Carol with a mixture of appeasement and defiance. 'Perhaps so, but knowing about things doesn't necessarily make you less angry. Your "feeling better" might also be a way of avoiding angry feelings ,' countered Dr L didactically, but not unkindly.,

Carol felt impotent and at an impasse with Dr L, and the two again lapsed into a silence, as long and uncomfortable as the one which had preceded it.

'I don't think individual psychotherapy would be suitable for you, but I'll see what the possibilities are for a group that you might be able to attend', opined Dr L: his magisterial manner indicating that their session and relationship were at an end.

Carol sensed, at that time, and a retrospective view indicates her correctness in this, that a group was not what she either needed or wanted. Carol's contact with the hospital was lost.

Carol was not 'damaged'in any obvious or dramatic way by the failure to develop any rapport with Dr L, but she reacted by developing a well-articulated suspiciousness of psychotherapy and its practitioners, which, at its sharper end, had a cynical and truculent edge. The blunter aspect revealed a wariness, more vulnerable and afraid. Her symptoms, so deeply rooted in her first and now current relationships, and her internal representations of these, continued a fluctuating but unresolved course. Only in recent times, after talking with me at length about her experience in particular, and the problematic nature of therapy and therapists in general, has she come to modify and destructure her mistrustful view.

Now, Carol is not the 'easiest' patient; often feeling threatened and hurt, she has developed a formidable capacity to distract by quips, intellectual commentaries and apparent 'insight' which, in fact, conceals from herself and others what she does not want revealed. These strategies were probably even more difficult to counter when Dr L saw her. But she maintains, and I believe her, that even ten years ago she might have been accessible to psychotherapy, had her interview been more geared to making contact rather than interpretations.

Let us shift our focus now from Carol to Dr L and construct a plausible, if hypothetical, understanding of what he was doing. The evidence, of course, is Carol's, but she is a reliable witness with a good memory and, most importantly, the pattern she describes is too frequent and significant for it to be glibly and technically dismissed, as merely a defensive manifestation of patients' difficulties; there is wisdom as much as hostility in the many bad (and good!) jokes about psychotherapists and analysts.

It seems that Dr L's style was prescriptive and didactic in its process. He presumed a well-defined and elaborated model by which to codify and 'understand' Carol's difficulty. So wedded was he to this model that it automatically led to a `technique', which he immediately applied; rather than slowly establishing a dialogue, he confronted her from the outset by the paradox of non-contact. The purpose of this, presumably, was to deprive Carol of her usual props and strategies, and via the ensuing anxiety to 'make her aware' of her fear, hostility, manipulativeness, or whatever. We may assume that Dr L was working from a psychoanalytic base, where he preconceived Carol's depression as being a consequence of retroflected anger, and that this anger itself is a residuum of her earliest developmental tasks of separating herself from mother, and integrating 'good' and 'bad' objects and feelings. Carol sees now that this kind of understanding has value in making sense of her turbulence, but is certainly not the only, or even the most effective, way of doing so. Other family and social factors have been equally important in leading Carol to her present conflicts and impasse. Dr L seems not to have heeded this, however. It is likely that he was a therapist of precise and rigorous training and strong conviction, who 'knew' what her psychopathology was, and the only effective therapeutic stratagem to be applied; all else would be an avoidance or dilution of these central truths. He did not, first, need to make a relationship with Carol, where he could learn about Carol's world in her own language. The important task was that Carol should learn from him, that he should demonstrate quickly and clearly to her the issues she must necessarily confront. He did not require much time to do this; his training had made him skilful and dexterous, and many of his colleagues admired and reinforced his articulate commitment.

According to Hannah Segal (1979), Melanie Klein believed that 'things cannot be a bit like this and a bit like that. In matters of science, there can be no compromise...'. While this may be a necessarily pragmatic principle in a Court of Law, where `truth' must be clear-cut and accessible to bureaucratic process, it is liable to become absurd or sinister when applied to situations that are as complex as understanding human nature. Those scientists concerned with the most precise observations and formulations – physicists – have long ago given up the search for inviolable truths. Since Einstein and Heisenberg (Einstein & Infield 1938) 'truth' has become relativistic and pragmatic; sometimes it is convenient to consider `matter' as a wave-form, at other times a particle – the 'truth' is either, neither, or both of these. The skill of the physicist lies in the sophistication and knowledge behind his 'juggling' with the different models.

In the realm of understanding ourselves and our fellows, this relativistic principle is even more important than in physics; our models may have a relation to truth, but they are not themselves 'true' in an immutable sense. We can introduce an illustration (Figure 1) here to clarify this theme:

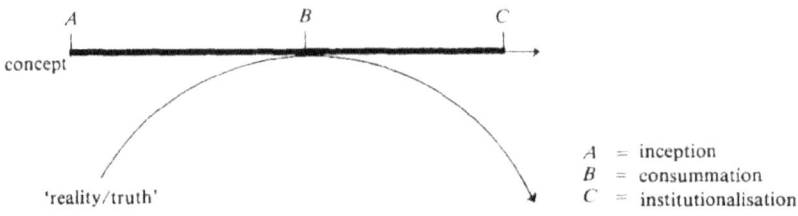

Figure 1. Concept and reality (The darker line, denoting 'concept', implies easier mental accessibility than the ultimately elusive, and fainter 'reality'.)

Notice here how the straight line 'concept' touches the curved 'reality' at only one point, *B*, but that further travelling along the concept departs increasingly from reality. Our psychological formulations often have this quality: we sketch a rudimentary idea, seeing a certain relation to reality, *A*; as we develop and refine the idea we reach an optimum point, *B*, of contact with reality, but further thinking along this line departs from it. The process of *A→B* is disciplined, creative and exploratory, but *B→C* is increasingly dogmatic, defensive and professionally solipsistic. It is part of the art of psychotherapy to know when 'point *B'* has been reached, or passed, and to consider another approach.

In academic and intellectual circles, ideas are often assessed by logical connection and coherence with other ideas. It is assumed that if a body of knowledge or theory is internally coherent, then it is somehow more true than one with internal discrepancies and contradictions. While such a philosophy has a certain aesthetic appeal, and may keep us in familiar territory, it is no test of the validity or usefulness of an idea. Eastern philosophies have long recognised the fruitfulness and wisdom in reconciling opposites and incongruents (ie Yin and Yang of Taoism). Another diagram (Figure 2) illustrates opposing concepts and their relation to reality. If we use this to survey psychotherapy, then concepts 1 and 2 would be closely related approaches, which are complementary and easily reconciled, unless they become institutionalised: an example of this would be Freudian and Kleinian Analytic approaches, both of which stress the importance of discovering or uncovering unconscious and archaic conflict.

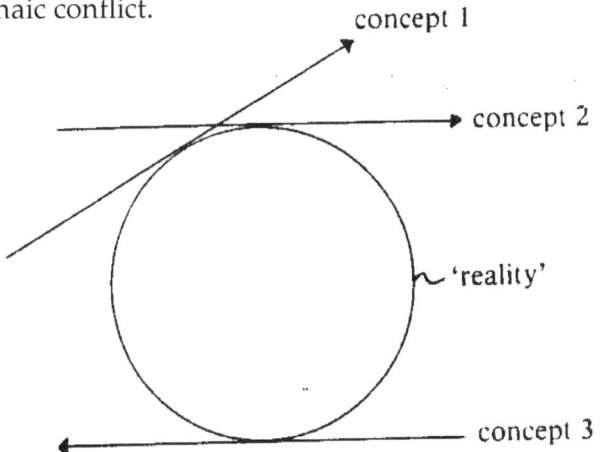

Figure 2. Complementary and opposing concepts and their relation to 'reality'

Concept 3, however, deals with aspects of reality in a way that is both juxtaposed and in the opposite direction; Glasser's Reality Therapy, which insists on personal responsibility in the present, and regards interpretation as likely to be an avoidance of this, represents such an opposing and incongruent concept. Although widely separated and having opposing vectors, concepts 2 and 3 come closer to resembling a circle than do concepts 1 and 2. Translated back to the realm of psychotherapy, we can see then that a therapist who discriminatingly chooses to work interpretatively from a Freudian base at one time, while at another will not do this but insists that the patient merely look at his actions and their consequences, is closer to the patient's reality (the circle) than the therapist whose eclecticism, for example, extends only to a choice of interpretative frameworks (concepts 1 and 2), or even more than the therapist who has only one conceptual system – his choice, then, is limited to how zealously to apply his technique. We can understand Dr L's professional behaviour as being an example of this.

'Scientific' studies in psychotherapy are concerned with the development of concepts from their inception (point *A* in Figure 1) to their consummation (point *B*). Tenacity to concepts beyond this point becomes an issue of institutionalisation or religious conviction, important phenomena which will be discussed later. The 'art' of psychotherapy may be thought of as the ability to draw different tangents at different times, to know when and how diverse forms of understanding and intervention may contact a patient's reality, and how these different lines may connect to make a whole (Figure 3).

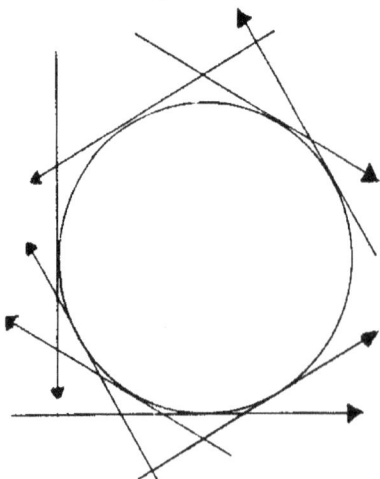

Figure 3. **Holism or eclecticism**

Such 'holism', of course, can never be complete, for it would require an infinite number of integrated approaches. However, a large part of our task in being a `good-enough therapist' consists in having competent and fluent use of a wide variety of ways of understanding. To evoke another metaphor, understanding people who come to us is like musical composition. The composer who knows about only one instrument will be restricted in the sounds he can create. The more he is acquainted with different, sometimes 'opposite', instruments and the relationship between them, the richer and more creative the music. Of course, the composer is thoroughly trained in the use of one instrument first, but it is the transposition of this discipline to other, less familiar, instruments and the learning of the new discipline of 'orchestral holism', which leads to the desired sound. Eclecticism in psychotherapy is often disparaged by more doctrinaire practitioners as being unformed, undisciplined and unfocused. I would maintain a different position: as with the composer, we must first learn one approach thoroughly, and then the fresh task of orchestrating the diverse and the unfamiliar awaits us. Our unwillingness to make this transition may lead us to the limited arena of expert, but stereotyped, performances: we may even institutionalise our performance, and validate our endeavours by having contact only with those professionals who agree with us. As with Dr L, though, we may develop skills much respected by our ideological cohabitees, at the price of relating to our patients with freshness and creativity; Dr L almost certainly had more rapport with his colleagues than with Carol.

It is not the psychoanalytic base of Dr L's practice that is in question here, but the fact that he seemed unable to part from it. With considerable sophistication he had turned a 'base' – which allows departure from it – into a 'trap' that does not, and to which Carol could respond only by acquiescence or struggle.

Such reductionism has earned mental health professionals the title of 'shrinks' who, by inference, reduce patients' human complexity, so that it may become subordinate to the professionals' sphere of influence and explanation. In this regard, psychoanalysis offers to such practitioners the same opportunities and dangers as other 'convergent' modes that have developed well-defined and elaborated systems of language, explanatory theory and professional protocol, for example traditional psychiatry. By contrast, those approaches, which are 'looser', more divergent and have less linguistic or conceptual precision, eg Existential or Client-Centred Therapy, would seem freer from this dilemma (though confronted equally by others). As in the realm of physical medicine, techniques and tools that penetrate, define and disable, however briefly, offer their potency inextricably linked with their hazards. Such activities require special capacities of discrimination and responsibility.

There arises also the important distinction between 'training' and 'education'. `Training', the more formal and didactic learning process, is almost certainly an important and elementary cornerstone in our development as therapists. The discipline involved in becoming thoroughly and systematically acquainted with one conceptual system is an essential requisite for later, more exploratory, ventures. Just as the infant needs a secure base in a consistent mother, to be able to leave her and relate to others and the vicissitudes of the wider world, perhaps therapists need a 'mother-model' which provides consistent familiarity, before the wider world of psychotherapy, with all its paradoxes, lacunae and frustrations can be confidently and creatively encountered. The process by which we venture away from the `mother-model', and make new and unforeseen contacts and syntheses, is our task of 'education'. There are other interesting and enlightening images we may draw from this metaphor; just as some children have a fearful and insecure attachment to mother, and cannot tolerate separation to make other relationships, so there are therapists who need always to cling to the mother-model, and respond with many kinds of anger or fear if this is challenged. As the mother-child relationship becomes fixed, so does the therapist-model relationship become institutionalised (as in Figure 1). Dr L probably represented this kind of petrified developmental arrest.

By contrast, the therapist who is able to internalise a good and consistent mother-model, and confidently but discriminatingly move into new and different therapeutic systems, is like the child who values and trusts his mother, but knows there are other good things for him in the world beyond.

'The will to truth is merely the longing for a stable world', Nietzsche (1888) wrote, many years before such matters became psychologically and academically scrutinised. His maxim is particularly relevant to those of us constructing (some might wish to say 'discovering') truths which we then apply to others. Many of us, perplexed and frightened by chaos both within and without, hope that some doctrine – religious, psychological, philosophical or political – will free us from this tempestuous burden. In recent times, the previously castle-like refuge of religious doctrine has crumbled, leaving psychology and politics, in particular, as ideological havens from a world that can otherwise seem frighteningly outside of our control, purpose and understanding. There are other quasi-religious functions involved: the formation of groups of fellow-believers can imbue members with a sense of mission, enlightenment and righteousness, making outsiders appear in darkest error. Viewed in this way, we can see why the definition and possession of the 'Right Way' in psychotherapy can be such a quirky, often jealous and paranoid business. It accounts also for Carol's first round of experience in this psychotherapy-roulette; she was dealing with Dr L's credo.

From the end of our intra-uterine life onwards, it is a central and never-ending task for each of us to learn to live creatively in the constant shadow of uncertainty. At our beginning, the womb expels us, the 'ideal' mother disappears or disintegrates, younger children unaccountably appear to supplant us. At the other end of our lives, our internal resources become erratic and fail us, friends and loved ones die, often without warning. In the middle is the swirling mosaic of choices, dilemmas and unfinished projects that make up the lot of Man in a rapidly changing world.

The task of tolerating and using uncertainty, to open up new possibilities, lies at the heart of sanity, growth and intimate relationships. Whatever formal diagnosis we apply to those who come to us, much of what we deal with are manifestations of disruption in meeting this challenge; we cling to archaic adaptations, notions, feelings and formulae largely because, whatever distress they may cause, they are ways of being that are relatively certain, familiar and predictable. A crucial part of our role as therapists then, if the patient is willing, is to beckon him away from his private but painful base of distorted 'certainty' and, in measures he can tolerate, introduce him to a more unpredictable world in which there are many more possibilities, both in how he perceives himself and how he may relate to others. An important practical question arises from this: how can the therapist who is anxiously and rigidly attached to his mother-model, help the patient abandon his subjective but 'certain' fictions, and journey out into a more real, but more uncertain, world?

True, there are equally vital and opposing tasks in psychotherapy. In some situations, if only for short periods, we need to operate with clarity, authority and a large degree of certainty. Just as children, at times, need a parent who is uncompromising and unswerving, so, of course, do patients. The therapist who is unable to do this when it is needed, faces similar long and short-term consequences as the parent who is unable to set firm, clear boundaries and rules. In taking this stance, however, we must satisfy ourselves that it emerges from a substantially considered choice, rather than our own incapacity to encounter the alien and the uncontrollable. Cleverness, often the product of training, is frequently and ritualistically overvalued in our professional culture, and then consists of pursuing a concept or ideology to the limits of sophistication and elaboration, giving an illusion of mastery and command over the unfamiliar.

Wisdom, the more delicate child of education, contrasts with, and departs from, such cleverness, and invites us, instead, to enter less charted areas, where the incongruous, the uncertain and the ungovernable await us, and our willingness to acknowledge them. It is perhaps a hallmark of maturity and substance in all our endeavours, to be able to make this kind of transition.

Ω

References

Einstein, A. & Infield, L. (1938) *The Evolution of Physics*. Cambridge: Cambridge University Press.
Nietzsche, F. (1888) *The Will to Power*.
Segal, H. (1979) *Klein.* London: Fontana.

Publ. in *British Journal of Psychotherapy*, Vol. 2(4), 1986

Three Types of Encounter in the Healing Arts

Dialogue, Dialectic and Didacticism

Western Medical and Psychiatric practice, anchored to its theoretical base of scientific determinism, tends to interventions that are administrative and prescriptive. This is derived from, and reflected in, the way in which knowledge is constructed, and the use of language. While this pattern of practice often works well in acute, circumscribed physical syndromes, it is usually far less effective when dealing with other, more frequently encountered, patterns of distress. In such situations the doctor needs to develop alternative ways of meeting and understanding his patient, which implies change in the 'metabolism' of language and knowledge. The discipline and discrimination involved in orchestrating these various kinds of encounter may give us a fresh perspective of 'holism'. A clinical case is described and a model presented to illustrate and amplify these principles.

`To think justly, we must know what others mean: to know the value of our thoughts, we must try their effect on other minds.'

William Hazlitt (1826), *On People of Sense*

`Mystification is the principal semantic tool of the would-be leader; demystification, of the man who wants to be his own master. Rousseau, Marx, Freud mystified; Emerson, Mill, Adler demystified. It is perhaps one of the immutable tragedies of the human condition that while the demystifier influences individuals, the mystifier moves multitudes.'

Thomas Szasz (1973), *The Second Sin*

Distress foreshadows and reflects fear and uncertainty in us all, and with it, to greater or lesser extent, the wish for the potent and protective figure or formula that will illuminate our way and absolve us the burdens of confusion, pain and the unknown. In our largest social groups we enact this in our choice (or extinction of choice) of political leadership, or legal and religious institutions. On our own, or in our most intimate groups, we devise more personal and idiosyncratic beliefs, rituals and protocols to ward off the potential storms or deserts of uncertainty.

Medicine and the healing arts span both these realms. At the public level, the doctor's white coat, his portentous professional institutions, and quasi-militaristic career structure all serve, in large part, to convey a variety of images, notions and experiences that create a sense of authority, confidence and safety. At a more private level, the doctor's use of technical language, and the way in which he makes physical contact with a patient, have the same psychological and social aims of ritualizing control, management and predictability. Such behaviours work best when they are harnessed to visible and effective problem-solving, such as an acute surgical emergency, but the further we depart from this type of situation, the more problematic this style of approach may become.

There are many kinds of distress which come to many kinds of healers where this type of structured and prescriptive manner becomes, at best, cumbersome, ineffective and insensitive, or at worst, infantilizing, insulting, injurious, and even corrupt by way of engendering unwarranted helplessness or damage in the recipient. It is, perhaps, the doctor's most challenging and unending task of self- education to discriminate when, how and to what degree to structure, define and manage what a patient brings to him in order to confer authority and predictability on the situation, and when, rather, to abandon such predication so that new forms of knowledge and interchange may evolve, which themselves spawn their own kinds of diagnosis and healing.

To understand more fully the roots and ramifications of these issues, we need to look at how we build up 'knowledge' and how this is transmitted or changed by the use of language. Both of these 'elements' — cognition and linguistics — are mechanisms underlying the more observable 'compounds' of patterns of practice that will be considered. For this reason a brief theoretical diversion is offered here to underpin considerations of language and knowledge that run as developing themes through this paper. It will be seen that such apparently 'academic' notions have an important, even determining, relationship to the important issues of dependency, autonomy, responsibility and awareness that many regard as crucial factors in healing and the maintenance of health.

Dialogue: the preliminary encounter

When any two individuals come together to relate and to communicate, each has his own 'framework of experience'. This comprises awareness of himself and the external world (percept); his ideas, theories or expectations concerning himself and the world (concept); and a feeling state accompanying these two (affect). Figure 1 illustrates this as a coherent system, the circle encompassing the triangle denotes the individual's framework of experience at the time of the interchange, expressed verbally in this kind of encounter in 'individual language', where each participant's utterances remain relatively uninfluenced by the other, and thus idiosyncratic.

In a 'dialogue', then, there is a free interchange of these components of experience, so that each will bring to the encounter elements of all three in his own manner, as a kind of exchange. Importantly, in the realm of dialogue, the experience and language of each participant remains autonomous of the other so that a 'free-trade' situation operates, as indicated in Figure 2. Note, also, that there is a distance between the two, which buffers each individual from any unwanted 'trespass', invasion or inclusion by the other.

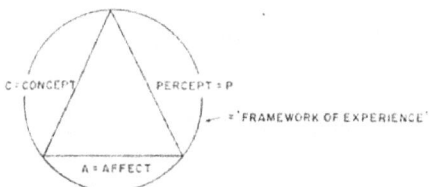

Fig. 1. The components of a participant in an interchange.

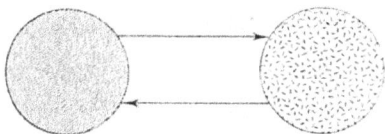

Fig. 2. Dialogue Free interchange of percept, concept and affect. Individual experience and language autonomous of the other.

There are, evidently, innumerable everyday examples of dialogue where individuals make contact in a manner that retains, intact and separate, the framework of experience of each participant. Let us look at how this operates in a typical and authentic medical situation.

Situation 1:

Mrs G, a recently widowed woman of 60, consulted her doctor, Dr H, about pains in her chest, particularly on awakening in the small hours of the morning, when she would become frightened by the unknown-ness of her distress and her alone-ness in having to endure it. She described her mixture of physical sensations (percept), the limited sense she made of them (concept) and the feelings which accompanied them (affect), while Dr H attempted to structure what she communicated to him and what he observed (P) by referring these to both the organizing concepts he had learned in his medical training (C) and, rather less, the feeling that arose in him during the consultation (A). He elaborated this process by asking her some routine questions about her chest pains and emotional state, and performing a physical examination. In attempting to fit all this 'information' about Mrs G into his professionally learned organizing concepts (diagnoses), the doctor became aware of his difficulty in this regard; he was most concerned about her heart, although some features were not typical of this source. The other categories that came to his mind focused instead on Mrs G's oesophagus or mind; in regard to the latter she had described to him her fear, and she appeared rather sad and tense. Dr H shared the dilemma arising from their dialogue, by saying 'Well I'm not sure what's wrong with you, Mrs G, I can't find anything on examination, but I think you should have some tests done at the hospital to see if there's any problem that I can't detect here, but which may need attention. I'll ask Dr J to see you.'

Let us stand back from this situation and see what has emerged. Mrs G and her doctor are in a 'free-trade' situation where they exchange unorganized 'bits' of experience, feeling or conceptualization, each with a different emphasis. The patient's main concerns and communications are of her disturbed bodily sensations (P), and emotional state (A); her ideas about these (C) are primitive and poorly organised. The doctor's focus is an attempt to form an organizing diagnosis (C), from what he observed and hears (P); Dr H did not pay much attention to the feeling of protectiveness and sadness (A) aroused in him by Mrs G's presence, he was too busy attempting to subsume Mrs G's story and their encounter to a well-defined form of his own thought and language (a medical diagnosis) which would transform the 'dialogue' into a form of 'didacticism', a form of interchange to be considered presently. His failure to do so urged him to refer the unfinished dialogue to Dr J, who, he hoped, would complete the transformation.

Didacticism: the organizing encounter

Situation 2:

When Mrs G went for her appointment with Dr J she was aware that she was going to a 'specialist'; someone who had greater effectiveness than her own doctor in defining the nature of her problem and what should be done. By the time she encountered him, she was apprehensive lest she was not able to give a clear and precise account of her problems; she felt awkward, too, in confiding in a stranger, particularly those fantasies and fears that so disturbed her in the early hours of the morning. Dr J greeted her in a polite, but busy and professional manner, getting quickly to the point of his many questions, which seemed both more numerous, organized and difficult to interrupt than those of her own doctor. Perhaps to her relief, he did not dwell on her emotional turbulence on waking, and passed quickly on to the questions concerning her physical symptoms. Mrs G then underwent a number of physical investigations which, the doctor explained, would help him locate the source of her pain. Dr J was, perhaps even more than Dr H, invested in doing this with speed and finality; he had spent many arduous years learning the required skills, and his professional status depended on his being seen to exercise them. He may have been a little dismayed, then, that Mrs G's physical examination, radiography and cardiograph were unremarkable, as he now had less definitive material with which to make his decision. 'I think your pains are caused by mild angina which isn't yet serious, and so isn't reflected in any of the tests', he explained to her, before elaborating the physical meaning of this, and the treatment he was prescribing for her. Mrs G's complaint was not typical of the diagnosis he made, but her answers to his questions suggested it as a real possibility, and Dr J thought it was too important a diagnosis to be missed. He 'discharged Mrs G back to her doctor', therefore, thinking he had defined the nature of her complaint and initiated a 'policy of management'.

As before, let us distance ourselves a little more from this situation and look at the emergent patterns. Mrs G's mosaic of physical sensations, thoughts and feelings has been sampled by Dr J, who has reorganized and redefined them according to his own method of perception (the physical examination) and conception (his deductive process of making a medical diagnosis). His own feelings while doing this were not within his awareness, partly because they did not fit into this way of 'diagnosing' a patient's problems. Mrs G came to the doctor with `dis-ease' which she expressed in her own language, but could find no personal meaning for; she leaves him with `disease' which is now expressed in the doctor's language, and to which he confers a meaning, which he must explain to her. Her own framework of experience with regard to her symptoms has become engulfed by the doctor's concept.

A consequence of her suffering from 'disease' rather than 'dis-ease' is that she can do little about it, except obey the doctor's instructions. It is as if her dis-ease, which has become transformed into disease, is now the doctor's property, though unfortunately residing in her body; he knows about it, defines it in his language, 'treats' or 'manages' or 'cures' the affliction, which she accommodates as an involuntary host. This process of 'didacticism' is illustrated in Figure 3.

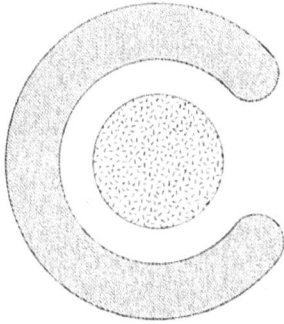

Fig. 3. Didacticism 'Take over' of experience, meaning and language of patient by the doctor.

Note that the 'Free-Trade' profile of the dialogue has changed into a 'take over', where one has 'engulfed' the other; the interchange now is not 'free', but organized and structured by one (the doctor), while the other (the patient), becomes a passive recipient. In the illustration, the patient is shown as being largely encompassed, which is true in a psychological and social sense as long as they are together, and is one of the most important features of this didactic approach. The patient here is protected and carried much as a kangaroo in its mother's pouch and, as in this analogy, it necessarily involves an abdication of autonomy, self-definition and self-determination on the part of one of the parties, while the other takes on these functions for the two of them. Didacticism is thus part of the way 'regression' and 'dependency' become organized professionally. Whether or not this is welcome, or ultimately advantageous to one, or other, or both parties is a complex issue which will be explored later. Clearly, if Mrs G, for example, was overcome with acute and severe chest pains and breathlessness, she would almost certainly welcome the opportunity to abdicate all responsibility for understanding or reacting to her experience while critically ill. On the other hand, the excessive or ill-timed use of didacticism will lead to unwarranted intrusion and control, with its later sequels of passivity, resentment and 'guerrilla warfare' of the psychological kind.

In Figure 3, which may illustrate Mrs G and Dr J, Mrs G is not totally encompassed, retains her own boundary and a space between the two. She still knows who she is, and can 'squeeze her way out' of this didactic arrangement if she so chooses. This is not so in extreme forms of didacticism. Within the healthcare field this would be illustrated by the critically ill patient in an intensive care unit who is physically encompassed by technology, or the institutionalized mentally ill who are contained and surrounded by a hospital environment. Such a situation is shown in Figure 4, and the analogy here could be made with the baby in utero; protection, enclosure and dependence are complete – there is little possibility here for the self's assertion or expression.

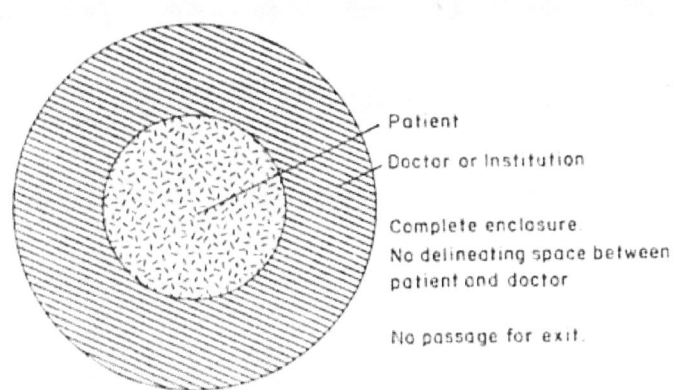

Patient

Doctor or Institution

Complete enclosure
No delineating space between
patient and doctor

No passage for exit.

Fig. 4.   End point didacticism.

Dialectic: the intimate encounter

Situation 3:

Mrs G was at first comforted and reassured by Dr J's authoritative and knowledgeable manner and the many tests he performed to see what was wrong with her. Unfortunately, the tablets he gave her didn't seem to make any difference to her symptoms, and her own doctor at first responded by increasing the dose, again without effect.

The next time she saw Dr H, he seemed less busy than usual, and Mrs G felt under less pressure to produce a rapid précis of her experience, so as 'not to waste the doctor's time'. Dr H, partly due to the reduced demands on him, felt fresher and more receptive than he had been when Mrs G had previously seen him and, as she walked into his consulting room, he paid attention to a sudden feeling of sadness arising in him, a tugging sensation located in his chest, as if she had brought the feeling in with her. In the wake of this clear but unexpected visceral signal, he recalled the death of her husband, Harry, six months previously – an event which he had heard about indirectly, and which, for some reason, had previously eluded his focus. When she went on to talk of her thoracic discomfort, he asked her to elaborate it in her own words: 'it's like a knot here' (rubbing the front of her left chest), 'as if there's something there that's going to burst, and then I go dizzy and feel I can't breathe . . .'.

Dr H then asked: 'When you lie awake at night, what do you think about?'

Mrs G's eyes moistened briefly, as she quickly looked up into the corner of the room, simultaneously biting her lower lip:

'Oh, I don't know . . . silly things, you know. It's difficult to say . . .'

Although not finishing her sentence, she looked at Dr H deliberately and directly, a desolate but tacit gaze.

Dr H paused a couple of seconds, sat forward a little closer to her, saying gently and tentatively: 'As you're talking, I have the sense that you feel sadder and more full of grief than you've conveyed to anyone . . . I'm wondering, too, about how much you want to say to Harry, about his leaving you, about being left on your own'.

Mrs G now sat forward, allowing herself to lean on the doctor's desk and saying: 'Oh yes . . . you seem to understand that. There's so much of it inside of me, pulling my mind in different directions; but I've always been one to keep a brave face . . . my daughters tell me I've been "wonderful" the way I've coped, and I haven't wanted to tell them just how bad I've felt, how lonely I feel . . .', she shrugged, as if discounting the interest of this to anyone but herself.

Dr H offered an image that surfaced and crystallised in his awareness: 'It's like you've had to deal, very much on your own, with two broken hearts; the one that killed Harry and the one that you're left alive with, that hurts when you're most alone in the middle of the night.'

'I don't know which I am; full of pain, hurting because I'm still alive when he's gone, or whether I'm just dead somehow, like Harry on the inside, although on the outside I'm just the same . . . can you understand that?'

'Yes, the broken heart that gave up, and the one that has to carry on painfully — it's like you have them both inside of you . . . it takes a long time for that kind of pain and emptiness to go away; to have your heart touched or warmed, so that you know you're alive, and you know you want to be alive. There are times when we have to die a bit first… to come alive again'.

'I think I've known that, at times, anyway, but it feels so much better just hearing you say it. It makes it more real somehow . . . like I know where I am and what I'm going through'.

Mrs G looked at the doctor sadly, but with less desolation than before; as if her heart was enlivened just a little already. The two of them sat together quietly for half a minute in a silence that was consummate and autumnal, as if they both needed a little time to digest, each in the company of the other, what they had produced together.

Mrs G, slowly straightening herself from the doctor's desk that she had been leaning against, gathered her coat and bag together, saying thoughtfully: 'I think I'll be alright, but it's hard. It's good to know you're here. Shall I come and see you next week, doctor?'

`Yes, I think you need to, and I shall want to know how you are', replied Dr H, aware of a glowing sensation in his chest. Perhaps his heart, too, so often numbed by business and his didactic functions, was beginning to warm.

Mrs G did return regularly for some months, but on a very different basis from before. Her chest pains became far less alarming for her and eventually disappeared without any further medical initiative from Dr H. She seemed to seek him out as a companion, helping her through a difficult passage; she knew that he could not take away her dis-ease, but he could help understand it, bear it and perhaps resolve it.

The doctor understood that his 'heart to heart' with his patient had eased the aching in her heart in a metaphorical and emotional sense; had this been reflected at a cellular level too? Dr H wondered. Was she now perfusing her heart when before she was, literally physically, blocking it off? In any case, the doctor mused, their encounter seemed to have penetrated beyond the reach of his medication.

The process and outcome of this last situation are clearly very different from the other two. Dr H did not here attempt to quickly subsume his patient's account of her experience to his own prior concepts, but allowed himself a period of uncertainty, where various notions and possibilities were invented in the moment and could be offered to Mrs G to sample, 'play with', explore, develop or discard as she wished. In doing this, the doctor paid equal attention to all the fragments of percept, affect and concept arising in both him and his patient; his own 'heaviness of heart' when she walked in the room was seen not as a contaminating influence to the medical interview, but as a potentially valuable emanation or expression which could be explored to find some kind of shared meaning. Likewise her involuntary physical reactions to his asking about her troublesome thoughts: when she turned her moistening eyes to the ceiling and bit her lip, Dr H had a new if tentative understanding of her – 'In her mind's eye she continually sees Harry; the sadness she experiences is beyond her capacity to tell the living. She searches for him with her eyes but bites her lip to stop herself speaking of this', Dr H had thought to himself, but also realized it was a subjective hypothesis to be offered to her to see if she would make sense of it. Mrs G. not only made sense of Dr H's metaphor of the 'broken heart', she elaborated on it, thus helping to create between the two of them a new and unique system of understanding, with its own symbols, metaphors and use of language. The physical movement of each toward the other physically, enacted what was happening at the psychological level; there was a convergence, even fusion, of their two worlds, so that the doctor's technical observations (P), his ideas about grief, body language, heart disease, ego-defence mechanisms and so forth (C), and the feelings arising in him (A), could be combined with the patient's disturbed bodily experiences and visual fantasies of her dead husband (P), her feelings of sadness and fear (A), and the notions she had about her physical disturbance and the life-passage she found herself in (C). The understanding that is constructed is new and unique and could only have arisen afresh in this situation; it could not have been organized or prescribed as a 'treatment'.

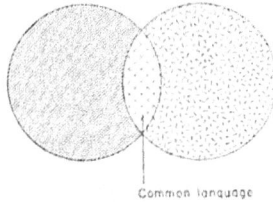

Common language

Fig. 5. Dialectic Fusion of framework of experience by two autonomous partners reflected in 'common language'. 'Merger' of experience.

Common language

Figure 5 illustrates this process of 'dialectic', where a 'common language' is created in the area of fusion of two individual selves and world experiences. This common language is made up of the two individuals, but transcends them both in creating something new. In many ways it is equivalent to sexual union where fusion and interpenetration leads to new life which is made up of, but transcends, the two participants. Using the economic metaphor again, dialectic is akin to a 'merger'. It is similar, too, to the psychoanalyst

Winnicott's[1] notions of 'playing' and 'intimacy' where these are considered as the creation and elaboration of a 'transitional zone' — a fertile area of interchange and improvisation between the self and the other. The fact that this dialectical approach involves a certain mutuality or intimacy, implies certain conditions, restrictions and prerequisites; it is only possible and only of value, for example, where both partners are prepared to abandon their own frame of reference and integrate it into something as yet unknown. It also implies a giving up of the 'control dimension' of the relationship, so that neither controls the other with regard to defining reality, using language, structuring the interchange, or prescribing what should be done. Clearly the didactic approach occupies the opposite pole from dialectic in these considerations.

This intimacy, necessary for, and generated by, dialectic is crucial to certain phases and aspects of healing. In situation 3, Mrs G had the sense of both understanding and being understood in a way that involved her own creativity and participation in the construction of the common language she achieved with her doctor. This being so, she felt empowered, dignified and compassionately accompanied in the experience, and enhanced in her capacity to clarify and express more. It is a fundamental psychodynamic principle that conflicts and dilemmas that remain unexpressed, unclear and unshared with others become amplified inside us and likely to become manifest in symptomatic difficulties. The act of understanding and entrusting our difficulties with another is often the first step in mastery and resolution. An important distinction should be made here between didactic and dialectic forms of insight and understanding. If Dr H had prematurely said to her: 'Part of your problem is that you have a masked depression. Your chest pain is due to you not letting go of Harry', he may have been correct and have been saying something similar, in content, to what he and Mrs G had arrived at in situation 3. However, this didactic insight would have been inflicted on her, and would be far less likely to be helpful; the essential processes of trust, rapport, mutuality and common language are missing, and Mrs G becomes, as she was in situation 2 with Dr J, the passive recipient of the doctor's organizing concepts.

The art of integrating science

Perhaps, though, Mrs G needed to pass through a phase where she abdicated any knowledge of, or responsibility for, her symptoms and be cared for and defined by an authority figure, as she was by Dr J In such a situation she may not have yet had the internal resources, or known Dr H well enough, to have entrusted him with the faltering first steps involved in self-exploration and intimate disclosure. In short, she may have needed `treatment' by Dr J's organizing scientific concepts – didacticism – as a necessary phase or 'regression' where she felt protected, unchallenged and unalone. Only later, with the passage of time and the development of dialogue with Dr H, could she go on to take some responsibility for, and see some meaning in, her symptoms. The shared development by which this happened – dialectic – passed from a 'treatment' to a `therapy' situation, where the doctor was more responsive to, but less responsible for, Mrs G. The framework of understanding, and the language used to achieve this, changed from the doctor's scientific ideology to an `existential' mode, jointly formulated.

Figure 6 illustrates the shifts involved in the three different kinds of encounter and the processes by which they occur.

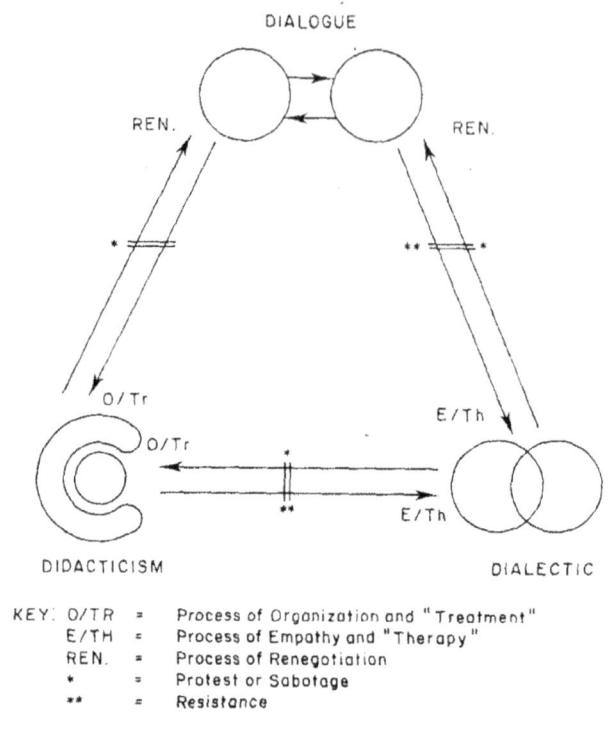

KEY: O/TR = Process of Organization and "Treatment"
     E/TH = Process of Empathy and "Therapy"
     REN. = Process of Renegotiation
     *   = Protest or Sabotage
     **   = Resistance

Fig. 6. The interpersonal dynamics of encounter.

Scientific medicine, as traditionally conceived and practised, involves a transmutation by the doctor of the dialogue he has with the patient, so that the patient submits to the treatment and abdicates responsibility for his distress. If either partner does not wish to continue this, or the treatment does not work, then, if the two wish to go on together, there must be a renegotiation through dialogue. If both are willing, able and motivated to find a more personal understanding and language for the problem, then there is a shift to a dialectic via the development of empathy. The naming of this change as 'therapy' (as opposed to 'treatment') implies the increased responsibility and activity of the patient. This can be abandoned by either renegotiation to dialogue, or reversion back to the treatment situation.

Where one of the partners wishes to change the form of the encounter unilaterally, without some readiness on the part of the other, then certain defensive or sabotaging strategies will be used by the one pressurized to change. For example, the doctor who makes a premature shift into didacticism by diagnosing, say, premenstrual tension, is unlikely to get the patient to take the medication as prescribed. Another common example of this is the patient labelled 'schizophrenic' who will not adhere to drug regimes. The psychiatrist might say – didactically – that the patient's noncompliance is part of his 'schizophrenic illness', but it may instead reflect the psychiatrist's personality and training whereby he is resistant to, or incapable of, meeting his patient in a dialogue or dialectic.

While 'protest' and 'sabotage' occur at largely conscious levels, 'resistance' operates unconsciously to defend a person against the authenticity, closeness and self-responsibility that ensue in any shift toward the intimacy of dialectic. Psycho-analytically, this term has traditionally been applied (didactically!) to patients, but it often works the other way round. Most hazardously in psychiatry, there is frequently a rapid moulding of a patient's communications so that they will fit into the doctor's diagnostic and treatment schemes; those that cannot be so tailored are either simply not heard or seen, or dismissed as lacking in 'clinical significance'. The fact that the doctor's didactic pronouncements and plans are often not effective may not lead him to renegotiating a dialogue, or attempting to construct a common language with his patient. In his own, and his profession's form of resistance, he may fall back even further into his didactic position by, for example, elaborating theories of 'psychopathology' of the patient's condition – an attitude and endeavour which may be institutionalized and applauded by his colleagues but, paradoxically, lead to increasing alienation from his patients. Such a doctor's investment in maintaining a didactic position is often based on a fear of the reverse; that he himself becomes the one that is dependent, turbulent, powerless or vulnerable.

Didacticism, at least while it operates, seems to confer immunity against such perils; the illusions, mechanisms and trappings of this have been dealt with in a previous article.[2] Even if the doctor is not resistant to shifting away from his didactic position, many of his patients will be. The investment in another person for certainty, the power of transformation, warding off dangers of the unknown in ourselves and the world around us may be an illusion, but a comforting one. Authoritarian relationships and institutions often provide, too, a certain security and familiarity. Freedom and autonomy are often too much of a challenge and a burden.[3] Thus, a doctor's attempt to provoke an unwilling patient to move away from their passive and defined role in the didactic arrangement will be met by some kind of sabotage or resistance. I remember a woman doctor who had been `treating', in an impotent and ritualistic form, a man for an endless stream of minor functional disorders, the favourite of which were 'sick headaches', for 15 years. He appeared, to the doctor, a stable, dull man whose lack of curiosity about the nature or meaning of his symptoms seemed part of his general passivity. One morning he came yet again, perhaps for the hundredth time, complaining in his stereotyped way of his inexorable complaints, asking:

'Isn't there something else you can give me doctor?'

'I wonder if there's something you ought to be giving yourself?', replied the doctor, for the first time attempting to break the pattern, she thought rather succinctly and profoundly.

He looked askance at her. 'Have you been on one of your new courses, doctor?', came the caustic retort, sly and rhetorical. She got the message, and he left with another prescription.

In this situation the patient clearly wished his doctor to assume a didactic role and 'treat' a 'disease'; he resisted any attempt she might make to destructure their familiar roles, so that he might become more self-governing, self-responsible or self-aware by exploring the basis of his dis-ease. He wanted to be a patient. It can be seen here how the doctor wished to redefine the problem existentially, while the patient wished to continue with an organic or deterministic approach to his problem. Here lies a central ideological distinction between the dialectic and didactic approach. Didacticism tends to scientific determinism and the notion of mechanical disease, which can only be cured by the expert. Dialectic is an activity arising from an existential outlook, with an emphasis on pursuing personal responsibility and creating personal meaning. Psychotherapy, an area whose psychological and social politics is quite as difficult as conventional medicine, has practitioners whose method is often dominated by one of these modes. The orthodox psychoanalyst, for example, works on the assumption that the patient's 'psychopathology' depends on unconscious processes that only a trained psychoanalyst can understand and treat; Freud himself talked of patients 'submitting' to analysis. Existential psychotherapists, in contrast, emphasize mutuality, authenticity, intimacy and the attainment of common language as being therapeutic; there is here no prescribed treatment or organizing technical language.

Clearly, in medicine, psychiatry, psychotherapy and all other forms of healing, we need to be able to shift with great dexterity between all three approaches with those that came to us. The skills of negotiating in dialogue, taking responsibility didactically, declining responsibility but allowing a new responsiveness in dialectic, are all cornerstones in the rich pattern of human intercourse that make up the healing arts. As in most other forms of intercourse, the problems arise when we are out of touch with one another's internal worlds, or wanting to interact in the external world in different ways. For the healer rigorously trained in the didactic sciences, it often requires a significant change and development of personality to foster equal skill in the artistic exercise of dialectic. The perennial and rather simplistic question: 'Is Medicine an Art or a Science?' can be reformulated more precisely and meaningfully by asking instead: 'How can we, with art and empathy, apply our medical science, and what is the science of applying this art and empathy?'.

It is hoped that this description of the three types of encounter provides some basis for an answer.

Ω

References

1. Winnicot, D.W. *Playing and Reality*. London, Tavistock Pubs., 1971.
2. Zigmond, D. 'Physician Heal Thyself: The Paradox of Wounded Healer'. *British Journal of Holistic Medicine,* December 1984. Vol 1: 63-71.
3. Fromm, E. *Escape from Freedom.* New York, Holt, Rinehort and Winston, 1941.

Publ. in *Holistic Medicine*, Vol 2, 69-81 (1987)

The Psychoecology
of Gladys Parlett

'Peace dies when the framework is ripped apart. When there is no longer a place that is yours in the world. When you know no longer where your friend is to be found.'

Saint-Exupery, *Flight to Arras* (1942)

Proud, elderly and sprightly, Mrs Gladys Parlett does not betray her inner burdens and chasms openly. Slightly tinted, sharply coiffed hair surrounds an alert, kindly, discreetly rouged face. Freshly pressed and quietly co-ordinated clothes accompany a manner that seems merely consonant and pleasant to the unwatchful. Those more canny might become aware of more disquieting signs; her tinted spectacles both frame and conceal restless and sorrowfully glistening eyes, white knuckles keep a grip on her handbag with primitive tenacity, her ankles lock together as if to prevent impulsive and involuntary movement.

Until her beloved George's death, Dr L.'s dealings with her had been infrequent, simple and matter-of-fact. To the doctor they had been undemanding, courteous and easy people, and his pragmatic contact with them reflected a cordial and uncluttered alacrity. Her bereavement, though, soon heralded an unprecedented change. She came to him frequently and with numerous and protean complaints; a previously dormant stratum of self now erupting with a lava of fermenting and inexorable dis-ease. Dr L., a busy practitioner, but not illiterate in the task of reading what is not directly conveyed, at first responded with familiar precedent, sympathetically and symptomatically. Her collage of headaches, giddiness, respiratory infections, arthritic pains and nausea received the kind of specific remedies that keep Dr L. in respectable, if undistinguished, company.

Recognizing that he was dealing with a woman, for all her years, unused to verbalizing her pain and conflict, he was patient and delicate in making deeper contact. She needed, he thought, much encouragement and support in clarifying and validating her underlying turbulence and sense of injury. He supposed, or hoped, that exposure and apposition, to himself, of her internal wound might guide her capacity for restoration. Exploring discreetly beneath her sense of physical peril and instability he suggested she take him into her gallery of memories; cherished sepia-like episodes and life-fragments, some idealized, many bitter-sweet, receding back to a post-Edwardian childhood.

Gladys, a middle child amongst many in a poor Methodist docker's family, perceived her world then as loving but harsh. She had few doubts regarding her place and role amongst others, but the conditions demanded of her for such kinship were strict and uncompromising. She grew shyly and demurely into a womanhood of loyal but limited bonds. She met George, a young docker, also in his early twenties, at a local wedding. He was then, and remained for nearly 50 years, with few deviations, a sensitive and steadfast companion. More socially confident than she, he provided through their long interdependence, both a bridge to, and a buttress against, the outside world's demands, vicissitudes and opportunities. By nature a retiring and retroflective person, she had, nevertheless, for several decades, a milieu in which she had an unquestioned, largely unconscious, sense of purpose and attachment.

No inconvenience to others

What is conveyed to the doctor now, though, are memories and vestigial fragments of Gladys's previous ecology. Her two sons, currently married, middle-aged and with their own families, have enacted with great success the aspirations of their prudent, once poor and conscientious parents: propelling themselves upward and outward in a society increasingly occupationally and socially mobile, they now occupy homes and work-roles beyond any experience or familiarity of their parents. Pursuing better employment opportunities, both sons have settled far from the declining and ghost-like community of the old docks. They are dutiful and attentive sons, reliable in maintaining contact by telephone, and driving the many miles from the salubrious suburbs to visit her. Sometimes from concern, sometimes through guilt, they wonder whether their stoic but hurting mother should live with one of them, but this possibility is fraught with practical difficulties — neither can offer a home capacious enough to provide Gladys with her own bedroom without depriving one of their children of theirs; an arrangement they perceive as erosive to their own family's ecology. Gladys, in any case, overtly and overly proud and self-sufficient, has pre-emptively parried, in many utterances, any arrangement where she feels she may be, as she puts it, 'a burden' or 'inconvenience' to others.

In Gladys's childhood it had been quite different, she remembers, for her own grandmother, Milly. That old lady, like Gladys, had lost her husband 15 years before her own death. But there were important differences. Milly remained very much at the centre of a large family which, through hardship, poverty and social inertia, had little opportunity for mobility, change and, therefore, disintegration. The old lady, the senior matriarch, living in cold, crowded conditions in the family home amongst three generations, was the repository of female know-how, oral family history and tradition, and, often with mollification, sometimes with contention, of counsel, judgement and verdict. Increasingly disabled with arthritis and lingering pulmonary consumption, Milly nevertheless lived out a frail yet powerful widowhood of central importance to those around her until her eighty-eighth year. Consulted for her experience of the tangible tasks of recipes or the management of childhood ailments, or the more intangible problems of how to find happiness, or at least peace, amongst others, Milly had little reason to think of herself as her granddaughter does; 'a burden' or 'inconvenience' to others.

Somaticized distress

Dr L, in his surgery and home-visits, spends much of his time attempting to decode, if possible detoxify, the somaticized distress of his many elderly patients. It was not always so. A young man when he first entered practice, intellectually crisp and eager to apply, directly and succinctly, the concise medical notions and tools he had imbibed assiduously in his hospital training, he found himself responding with a polite, brisk veneer which masked an intense irritation when he encountered those, like Gladys Parlett, who somehow defied his efficient and medically rigorous ministrations. Like a sheep dog he would, with energy and vigilance, attempt to round them into his pen of medical diagnoses and managements only to find, repeatedly, that his 'good work' was to no avail. Many of them, with apparent obstinacy or perversity, didn't follow his instructions, developed side-effects to his prescriptions, wouldn't give up the medley of their complaints and symptoms. `If it weren't for these damn patients, I could be a good doctor', retorted a wry and weary older partner when the young Dr L sought commiseration and advice for his increasingly chronic sense of frustration and impotence. `Frankly, when I see them coming through the door, the question I ask myself is "How can I get them out as soon as possible?"', was his senior colleague's acid and nihilistic counsel.

It was some years before Dr L could understand and make creative use of these feelings of redundancy and defeat, to realize that this somehow mirrored his patients' experiences of decline, abandonment and nullification. He had, first, to face his own losses, witness his parents become elderly, and sniff his own mortality and transience. Dr L's private struggles and dilemmas in this arena have slowly transformed his way of understanding and responding to these refractory and disequilibrated people. He sees now that this public role as a family doctor has a symbolic significance for them, far more subtle and demanding than the problem-solving, technically-based functions in which he had previously immured himself. From a world rotating and changing increasingly rapidly around a technological axis, those at the periphery, particularly the elderly, unplaced and unable to contribute, are thrown off by a kind of social centrifugal force to become society's 'loose-bodies', disconnected and disinherited.

Gladys's grandmother, Milly, was part of the Stream of Life until her own death. Gladys, in contrast, must face her involution and ending, unaccompanied by the evidence of fresh life, the tending of which is one of the few things to make approaching death meaningful and bearable. Human contact and nourishment, having a social role in which we find meaning and which is valued by others, are the social prerequisites for inner and outer peace.

Gladys, and so many of Dr L's elderly 'regular attenders', have little such social role, contact and nutrient to sustain them. Their dis-ease, for them often ineffable and intense, finds inchoate articulation in their bodies. Sometimes, with encouragement from Dr L, there can be a translation into words. At other times this seems pointless and unnecessary, and a tacit understanding grows implicitly. Dr L has come to recognize the symbolic, perhaps unconscious, investment that is made in him and his surgery-environment. The waiting area is often a kind of village square where the elderly and isolated are, for a while, part of the milling of a local community; familiar faces encountered, fragments of gossip exchanged, babies paraded, admired and envied, older children reprimanded and humoured. The doctor's room becomes a sanctum or retreat where secrets, pains and private burdens may be, if only briefly, unloaded, alluded to and shared.

Dr L's physical presence, reassuring in its familiarity and constancy, has great importance for those whose personal landmarks have gone, receded or become rare and ritualistic.

For those seldom touched, the physical examination becomes imbued with potent ingredients of care and recognition, something that eluded his earlier judgement when such activities were determined more rigidly by 'clinical indications'. Any medicines he may prescribe, too, have meaning and functions he would have overlooked before he came to understand the anguish that can he born of aloneness. The bottle of medicine or tube of cream becomes a kind of talisman or reminder of the doctor's continuing existence when he is absent.

A waiting room for death

Gladys Parlett's anguish and sense of desolation have been intense and profound and, at times, beyond the reach or influence of Dr L's empathic interest or rationalized medications. One week she sat, almost immobile and mask-like, and talked obliquely, with a darkly-veiled foreboding, of ending her life. Managing for the first time to persuade her to see a psychiatrist, he arranged an appointment for her to see a consultant known to him as an approachable, sympathetic and psychologically skilled practitioner. This initiative was curtly and bureaucratically rebuffed. A phone call from the outpatient secretary indicated that all patients of her age had to be seen in the Psychogeriatric Unit; no exceptions could be made. Dr L balked, complied and acted accordingly.

The psychogeriatric young registrar pronounced the old lady 'significantly clinically depressed' while also surveying her isolation and 'vulnerable, insecure personality that has led to her notable lack of confidence and tendency to depressive illness since the loss of her husband . . .' A change of antidepressant medication and attendance at a Geriatric Day Centre 'for support and socialization' were recommended.

Much to Dr L's disappointment, but little to his surprise, Gladys developed intolerable 'side-effects' to both the chemical and social prescriptions and discontinued both. It was difficult to assess the possible physiological basis to her reaction to the drug, but her intense dislike of the old people's Day Centre was more easily understood: 'It's like a waiting room for death' she said with a stark, ruthless economy that arrested Dr L's breath for several seconds. 'They're very nice there, very kind, but I don't want to sit around with all those old people that I don't know, being "jollied along" . . . I know you don't have much time, doctor, but I'd rather come and talk to you, it's more natural, more like real life . . . I've known you and Sheila [the receptionist] for years, so it's like family, if you know what I mean. I hope you don't think I'm being difficult.'

Many might have done; Dr L did not, though the task of surrogate kinship, he reflected, was paradoxical in its ordinariness and complexity.

Separation from life's flow

For a profession currently festooning itself with variations on the themes of 'holism' and 'community care', people like Gladys Parlett confront us with daunting and growing challenges. By well-rehearsed rote we are liable to ascribe her distress to some type of psychiatric phenomenology or psycho-pathology, thus deflecting from a perspective which sees her disintegration as an individualized microcosm of a dislocation and decay happening increasingly in our socially fragmented times. Gladys's symptoms can, perhaps, be most clearly understood in terms of her growing and profound alienation from those around her. She is deprived of social function, substrate and network.

Milly, through a long, often cruel and tragic life, never lost a sense of belonging and purpose amongst others. Gladys, by contrast, in a life increasingly free of the kind of violent vicissitudes, thraldom and injustices her grandmother was subject to, enters her last stretch without this essential *raison d'être.* Her life now lacks an 'existential holism'. Her anguish flows from not being part of the Whole. Dr L, whose waiting-room bustles with human traffic, whose familiarity brings continuity, whose words and touch imply knowledge and interest in her private world, provides a sadly sparse but cherished sense of contact and inclusion. Despite its assigned function, the Geriatric Day Centre was perceived by Gladys as being a form of caring which separated her from the rest of humankind.

There is a certain irony and paradox in treating Gladys Parlett within the special designation of 'psychogeriatrics'. Certainly, her intense misery and despair warranted more time, attention and facilities than Dr L could muster but, as she made trenchantly clear, she could not tolerate this in a form which underlined her separation from life's flow. With the solid but spurious logic of our times, we assume that a growing problem must be given special and separate facilities, practitioners and premises. But if Gladys is to be reinstated into any Family of Man it makes little sense to attempt this in a manner which purports to create a 'community' comprised solely of the aged. The meaningful and healthy ecology of the aged cannot evolve from isolation. It must include the young.

Among the intriguing and tragic perversities of the human condition is the fact that the most enduring and certain of our bonds arise in the midst of hardship, adversity and common struggle. There were few lonely and alienated people in the last World War. When we are not engaged in the struggle to survive we are occupied by the task of creating personal and social meaning. The burdens of (relative) peace, prosperity and proliferation of choice may be often unacknowledged, but are inescapable. In an age where it has become the desired norm to define and pursue our own *modus vivendi,* where technology both generates and catalyses social diffusion and mobility, it is difficult to keep crucial events of our life-cycle within a familiar and ecological human matrix. The hospitalization of birth, decline, grief and death are all, to some degree, indices of our failure to live 'holistically' with one another.

As our real community dwindles, and neighbours become strangers, family becomes (albeit loyally) nostalgic visitors, the church is vandalized and empty, and the corner-shop closes down, we create fictional or symbolic substitutes. Perhaps television's *Eastenders* and *Crossroads* and the doctors' new ideologies of *Therapeutic Communities* and *Community Care* are akin in their efforts to provide 'societal prostheses', devices that provide, by artifice or illusion, a sense of community when the natural community is perishing. Gladys's shrill protest about the Day Centre, a kind of phantom-limb pain, alerted Dr L to her defiance of the alien and the unnatural. Holism, he has come to recognize, extends tantalizingly and without limit beyond the simple and tidy notions he had assembled and displayed, Lego-like, in order to become a doctor.

Publ. in *Holistic Medicine,* Vol. 3, 9-14 (1988)

The Front Door of Psychotherapy

Aspects from
General Medical Practice

'He who knows others is learned
He who knows himself is wise.'

Lao Tse (6th century BC), *The Character of Tao*

'It is far more important that one's life should be perceived than it be transformed; for no sooner has it been perceived than it transforms itself of its own accord.'

Maurice Maeterlinck (1896) *The Deeper Life, The Treasure of the Humble*

Healing and growth, through the exploration and expression of the hidden inner-world, is certainly as old as the written word, and probably as ancient as the earliest forms of communication of abstract thought. The last few decades have seen a rapid and diverse organization of such quests, in the form of 'psychotherapy' in its many guises. What these variegated and sometimes discordant schools have in common is the point of departure: the person seeking psychotherapy is already consciously committed (albeit ambivalently!) to the task of expanding their realms of self-awareness and self-responsibility. All such people may be said to commence from the 'lobby' of psychotherapy.

The General Medical Practitioner, however, is faced with very different, though related and equally challenging, psychological and existential tasks. Those who come to him for help are often unaware, or denying, of how their physical or mental dis-ease may derive from their on-going conflicts and dilemmas, and thus see any affliction or help as coming from outside their personal sphere of influence, awareness and responsibility.

The doctor's opportunities and challenges thus occur at the 'front door' of psychotherapy and it is always uncertain whether or not the patient will wish to enter. The doctor's role of 'doorman' here is a complex and interesting one, demanding much in the way of tact, timing and imagination, all of them skills particular to the setting. Unlike the professional psychotherapist, he has often had a long, punctuated and varied contact with the patient, often at crucial life-events, and this can offer him a vantage point and informal, though powerful, rapport that is unique.[1] The following descriptive and narrative case-histories or scenarios illustrate not only the problems of dealing with 'psychosomatic' syndromes which may be construed as the doctor's special territory, but more generally with the 'elements' of psychotherapy which underlie every genus of verbal healing.

Case No. 1:
Clarification or exorcism? Very simple psychotherapy

Mrs R seemed edgy and truculent when she entered Dr S's consulting room. Amanda, her four-year-old child, looking frightened and bemused, was thrust sharply towards Dr S. as an accusatory portent, an Item of Evidence for the Prosecution. Amanda stood with pale and compliant immobility as her mother quickly and purposefully unbuttoned her daughter's blouse, to reveal a small annular lesion on her chest, which the doctor immediately recognized as Tinea. He sighed privately with relief; he had expected something far worse.

'It's only Ringworm, Mrs R. Nothing to worry about. I'll give you some cream to apply, and it will clear up very quickly.' Dr S averred with bright and brisk reassurance.

Both his conviviality and authority were unexpectedly assailed:

'That's exactly what you said last year, but it's back again', retorted the flushed and angry mother, disconsolate and her eyes beginning to brim with hapless tears.

Dr S sighed again, now less privately and with the exasperation of a busy man obstructed. Biting back a mounting petulance, he struggled to retain a courteous image of helpfulness.

'Look, Mrs R., Amanda's skin has got a small Ringworm infection, that's all. It will soon clear up, even if she has had it before. But I don't understand your anxiety about all this – there seems to be something else that's bothering you that I don't know about…'replied the conciliatory doctor, now feeling as bemused as the silent and compliant small girl between them. It seemed to him that the mother had her own private, and as yet indecipherable, agenda, and he needed her to share this with him.

'It's all very well for you to say that, doctor, but what am I to think when she's full of worms…?' exclaimed the preoccupied mother.

'Worms!! Ah! I see …' exhaled the doctor, a sense of benign command returning with a fresh and growing comprehension of this uneasy and cramped impasse.

'Yes, doctor. She can't go on like, this with worms inside of her. … it can't be good for her…' continued the pressured Mrs R., hoping that enough leverage against the doctor would somehow rid her daughter of this largely invisible pestilence.

The doctor was now quick to understand and salvage the dialogue that had so nearly foundered from the mother's misconception, arising from the colloquial misnomer of this superficial yeast infection, Tinea corporis. Mrs R., witnessing her doctor's fresh comprehension, was now receptive to his explanation and reassurance. She softened and listened, the colour returned to Amanda's cheeks and Dr S stopped his impatient sighing. Their departure was one of tacit affection, peppered with jokes and reciprocated apologies. The doctor later that morning shared his story over coffee, an offering of comic relief, with his fatigued and embattled partner. It could, he realized, have turned out very differently.

What Dr S had here achieved with Mrs R. cannot be called 'psychotherapy' in its more formal sense, and yet the successful outcome of this short, highly-charged and rapidly shifting interchange depended on principles of communication and response which are cornerstones of psychotherapy at all levels of intensity and complexity.

The doctor had first to listen and observe afresh – the mother's shrill and remonstrative manner clearly conveyed much beyond the small, harmless lesion presented, and he had thus to consider that the meaning of the 'Ringworm' had very different connotations to himself and to his two frightened patients. It was only by allowing a hiatus in the usual structure of his interview, that Mrs R.'s fantasy or misconception of worm-infestation, her 'internal reality', could be crystallized, communicated and understood. Only then could both patient and doctor arrive at a new understanding of one another.[2]

Had Dr S needed to be in control at every stage of the interview, and forged ahead uncompromisingly with his initial frame of reference and didactic reassurance ('Nothing to worry about Mrs R., just use the cream ...') all three participants in this transaction would have left with further difficulty in store: Dr S would have gone home with a headache from frustrated ingratitude, Mrs R. and Amanda a symbiotic complex of anxious and unattended dread, coupled to an increasing mistrust of their conscientious but harassed doctor.

The medical prescription, the fungicidal cream, would be an adequate antidote to the physical lesion, but it was the development of understanding in the relationship that healed the growing emotional lesion. Mrs R.'s gruesome misconception – of 'Amanda being full of worms' – seemed to the doctor fortuitous, and due to misconstruction from the oddly termed 'Ringworm'. His task of exorcizing this damaging notion was thus much simpler and swifter than the psychodynamically generated complexes that challenge the skills of the psycho-therapist or analyst. Had Mrs R.'s fantasy of worms arisen instead from deeper, perhaps unconscious compounds of guilt, nameless dread, and inchoate destructiveness – the elemental stuff of psychoanalysis – she would not have departed as easily and lightly as she did, and would surely return with other tense and tangled communications.

Case No. 2:
Inner and outer listening: emotional literacy

A large and plethoric man, Mr B. looked briefly and searchingly toward Dr C, smiled nervously, moved away, and then shifted his doleful, heavy frame back toward the doctor.

Dr C, realizing his patient's first utterances would be difficult and important, put down his pen and sat back quietly.

'Doctor, I think I'm an alcoholic ... well I know I'm an alcoholic, I suppose. I know you can't do anything about that, so I'm probably wasting your time ... I just thought there might be something...'

Several routine questions offered to retrieve the fading Mr B. revealed to Dr C the severity and pattern of retreat into the haven of alcoholic oblivion in this unhappy and anxious man. But it was Mr B.'s underlying unhappiness itself, rather than a medically precise definition of his alcoholic abuse, that the doctor gently probed towards:

'Most people who have your kind of difficulty are attempting to get away from a feeling, or a situation, that is difficult or painful for them to manage or put into words, and I have the sense that's so with you, Mr B.', proffered the doctor, in a tone inviting but, he hoped, unintrusive.

'Yes, that's true. I do most of my drinking when I'm upset and all churned up. I think I can't stand all this aggravation, I want "Out", and then start drinking', elaborated an alert and engaged Mr B.

Dr C usually found himself pessimistic and patronizingly 'tolerant' with alcoholics, who, in his experience, seemed to have more guile in dissembling their problem, than he had talent or commitment to intervene in any way that might be hopeful or helpful. But Mr B. was a disarming and refreshing contrast in his candour, and the transparency of his underlying difficulties.

'I have a sense of you as being easy-going and genial on the outside, but hiding your hurts, grievances and resentments inside, where no one can see them ... so that there's a big gap between how people see you and what's really going on inside of you, and that gap makes for a lot of loneliness and fear ...', Dr C suggested, attempting to integrate his own experience of Mr B. with what Mr B. was saying about himself.

'Yes, that's just how it is ... there's this whole other side of me, like a small kid that's really angry and unhappy, and doesn't know what to do...'

'And drinks as a way out?' the doctor suggested before hearing more specifically of Mr B.'s lifelong difficulty in facing conflict and 'aggravation'.

The only child of an unhappy and tense union between a timorous, phobic mother and domineering, bullying father, he had learned early to survive by obedience, almost to the point of invisibility. But such early survival strategies, now fixed and long outmoded, had long ago rendered Mr B. mute in the face of challenge, passive in his needs, and emotionally inarticulate in his closest relationships. It did not surprise the doctor to learn that Mrs B. reacted to her husband's stalwart but hurt silences by bullying provocation, in an exasperated effort to create some sense of contact and definition with her sullen and inscrutable partner. The fact that her attacks led only to his further retreat into the morass, accelerated by his drinking, did not lead her to abandon her pattern, but amplify it.

In this first, and a later, longer interview the doctor gently guided this perplexed and hitherto inarticulate man in his efforts to make sense and connections, amidst the cycles of impotent resentment and retaliatory and palliative drinking. Thus encouraged, Mr B. took up the doctor's suggestion of seeking further counselling.

'I'm not drinking at all now, doctor', reported a direct and proud Mr B., and when the doctor asked him how he saw these first important steps of mastery, the reply was of great interest and edification to Dr C.

'When I first came to see you I thought you'd have little time for me, tell me to stop, that it was my problem and I was damaging myself – that sort of thing. That's what I expected, and I knew it wouldn't help. But you did something quite different: you really listened to me, and thought carefully about what I said. That hadn't happened to me before, and it's very important because it's started me listening to, and thinking about myself. With my counsellor now I'm beginning to see all sorts of things that I'd spent years running away from. I'm really pleased I came when I did.'

Dr C was pleased, too; it is not often that a patient comes to him in such a state of readiness to express and explore the underworld of conflicts and dilemmas, that are essential for radical and healing changes in the attitudes to oneself and relationships to others. The doctor had read much psychiatric literature concerning the efficacy or viability of psychotherapy in different clinical syndromes, suggesting that it is the clinical diagnosis which will determine the outcome of such endeavours. Such 'scientific' formulations never appealed much to his more humanistic temperament, and as the years have gone by he has been more impressed by determinants that can be more ordinarily expressed.

The capacity for candour, courage, curiosity and contact – both with what is within oneself and the other person – have seemed more accurate indicators of a healing dialogue. With many of his patients suffering from 'minor' neurotic complaints, he has never, despite his best efforts, been able to find a way through to these health-generating qualities: his words and attentions seem to bounce back at him. Others with more 'major' psychiatric stigmata, which numerous learned and specialist tracts would deem unsuitable or unlikely recipients of verbal healing, have surprised and inspired him with their readiness to enter the cauldron of challenge and change.

In these many journeys and encounters he has come to a new understanding of the word 'encourage' – as a young practitioner his encouragement consisted of convivial utterances designed to 'make the patient feel better', or at least appear grateful, if only for short periods. Fostering and nurturing the courage that inspires all health and growth, a more literal and substantial 'encouragement', had taken years of his own inner struggles and searchings to develop: encouragement must arise from a position of resonance, not rhetoric. We heal from our own healed wounds. [3, 4]

In parallel with Dr C's growth of understanding of encouragement has been his perception of 'emotional literacy' as a core element in health, growth and psychotherapy.[5] To remain 'in balance' with ourselves and others we need to be clear about our feelings; to name them, to read them, to articulate them. Without this emotional literacy there can be no solid sense or affirmation of the Self, from which any meaningful negotiation or mutuality with others becomes possible.

Mr B. was suffering from such illiteracy; raised in a family where needs and feelings were persistently distorted and discounted, he grew into a man effectively mute and affectively stunted. His alcoholic balm, intended to ease the pain of alienation from himself and others, only deepened the chasm. Many patients, it seems to Dr C, consult him because of such patterns of the inchoate and ineffable. With Mr B. it was his behaviour that led him to seek his doctor's counsel, but more often it is the patient's body that signals and expresses such dis-ease and disequilibrium. The doctor's task is then clear, but often difficult, in helping his patient in the reclamation and deciphering of their disowned and neglected Self.

The long abandoned term of 'Alienist' for what we now call the Psychiatrist – a title connoting the re-engagement of those afflicted by alienation from themselves and others – seemed to encapsulate much of what Dr C must achieve in any healing endeavour with his patients. The doctor, though, is mindful of how demanding this is of the practitioner: as his use of 'encouragement' reflected the painful growth of his own courage, so his efforts at fostering 'emotional literacy' in his estranged patients could only parallel his own capacity for emotional clarity and articulation. To hear others we must listen to ourselves.

Case No. 3:
Feelings as wounder, feelings as healer

Dr T was only outwardly acquainted with Bill, an angular wiry man in his mid-fifties with an air of contained and circumspect vulnerability, and when he came with a recent exacerbation of his duodenal ulcer, the doctor wondered what had rekindled this invisible and self-generated wound. Prefacing his tense, though not unpleasant, communications with self-discounting apologies for bothering the doctor, Bill appeared to regard his hurts and needs as being unworthy of others' attention and care. A Council gardener in a small and meticulously tended local park, this well-regulated and compliant man always attended an evening surgery after his day's work, attired in his regulation green overalls.

From previous contact, Dr T had been witness to his limited but loyal life: his father dying in wartime combat, an only child, he had lived with his mother in their small late-Victorian flat until her death five years previously. Her demise had been slow and demanding, and he nursed her throughout this long and gruelling decline with fierce but quiet dedication, parrying any suggestion of her 'going away' to hospital. She died at home, a task painfully and painstakingly completed. When, some months later, Bill had requested an embrocation to soothe an overworked muscle in his thigh, a casualty of his silent and earnest training for the Marathon, Dr T mused on how, symbolically, his stoic self-sacrificing relationship with his beloved mother had been soon replaced. The doctor, while dealing with the matter of Bill's strained muscle, recalled with poignancy the title of an old black and white film: 'The Loneliness of the Long Distance Runner', but Bill's manner then had seemed dour and uncompromisingly matter-of-fact. The doctor did not share his image.

On this occasion, though, Bill seemed softer, and the doctor felt less prohibited from approaching his personal World, and when Dr T carefully asked him if there was anything in his recent life that had opened up his old internal wound, Bill's jaw trembled, his sinewy, tight-body sagged and he wept the copious, ancient tears of a man released from a long imprisonment.

'It was Frank going like that ...' he sobbed, attempting to stem the tears with a peremptory and remonstrating hand. 'He was my best mate. There was nothing the matter with him, but he just went... just went.'

From Bill's spontaneously articulated fragments of narration, and from his own delicately interposed questions, Dr T was able to assemble something of the significance of this much beloved and irreplaceable companion. Frank, another single man of similar age, had worked alongside Bill for a decade in the small and intimate park that had become a kind of child for these two childless men. Frank, apparently healthy and sanguine, had collapsed and died, at the verge of a flower bed, suddenly and without portent.

Bill was able to command back his tears and create a brave, red-eyed hiatus as he shared with the doctor something of his cherished friend and the painful void his sudden departure had left. As Dr T understood, more than ever before, the fragile and lonely courage lying behind the rather impassive exterior, Bill convulsed with another involuntary wave of recent and archaic grief. Dr T sat touched, attentive and silent, feeling like a mother cradling an anguished infant.

'I'm sorry, doctor to be like this… it's stupid, a grown man like me crying like a baby…', a finger and thumb pressed tightly and censoriously to his eyes, a vain attempt to enforce his usual containment.

'Not at all', Dr T uttered softly. 'I'm sad with you that you have this pain and grief, but very pleased you're able to share it with me; that's not at all "stupid". There are times for all of us when we need to cry and be cared for by others. I've long had a sense of you as being both courageous, but very hard on yourself in this way; that you won't allow yourself these very natural and human needs. I'll give you some tablets which will help cure your ulcer but, you know, what you've started here with me, sharing and expressing your feelings, may be the best medicine you can give yourself. I know it's hard and strange for you, but it's something I'm more than willing to help you with if you wish. It can be a great comfort, to have a safe place to talk about things that are kept hidden in other relationships in your life. I don't want to intrude, but I'm here to listen if you want me.'

'Yes, I do see what you're saying … and thank you, doctor. It's good to know you're here'. Bill replied, his voice more sonorous; a quiet, economic and characteristic coda.

Dr T remembered from his earlier training, reading long and complex treatises on which, among the innumerable physical ills to which the flesh is prey, were thought to be 'psychosomatic', and what the diseased part was symbolically, unconsciously, but precisely expressing and enacting.[6] Dr T's view has evolved into something rather more ordinary and less scholarly, for it has seemed to him that any illness can signify the discordance, the 'unfinished business',[7] the mere unhappiness of its host, and that the important question is not 'Is this illness "psychosomatic"?' but 'How may this person's inner and relationship life contribute to their illness, and (how) can I usefully and tactfully intervene?'[8] Aware, too, of the growing research on how immune and repair systems in the body reflect unexpressed and unresolved feeling,[9] Dr T has now a far wider perspective of how the expression of hidden and trapped feeling is so often crucial to recovery and the maintenance of health: Bill's expulsion of painful and palliating tears, a 'natural' therapy, are quite as important as the synthetic compound the doctor gave him to quell the acid production in his stomach. Such is 'Holistic Medicine'.

But there is more to this 'in vivo' psychotherapy than mere catharsis; for Bill may learn, through his experience with Dr T, that he can share powerful feelings with others, that both can survive it, and that from these a new growth and modus vivendi becomes possible. Whether or not he takes these tasks into the more deliberate territory of 'in vitro' counselling or psychotherapy, he has encountered, in its humblest form, what the psychoanalyst Michael Balint terms 'a New Beginning'.[10] While the doctor's interest, skill and 'encouragement' are clearly important in these first steps of encountering such challenges, it is ultimately Bill's own capacities of courage, curiosity and candour that will decide how far through this 'Front Door of Psychotherapy' he decides to travel and explore.

Case No. 4:
Being there

It was an exceptional and dramatic illness that Alice had suffered when vacationing with her husband and two teenaged sons in a West Country resort. A detailed hospital letter, replete with technical details, chronicled how she had, from apparently good health, almost died from a rapidly spreading perineal infection which, within twenty-four hours, had spread to her blood-stream, rendering her comatose and moribund, to be plucked from death's door by the vigilant dedication and expertise of the Intensive Care Unit. A horror and a miracle, Dr D had thought as his eyes scanned the scores of investigations that had guided the medical salvation of Alice, but which left

Dr D perplexed and ignorant as to why Alice had been so savagely felled in the first place.

She had rarely seen Dr D, and when she entered his room looking pinched, tired and grey, his attention was focused almost solely on the physical ramifications and sequelae of her nearly fatal complaint. An examination revealed a small residual abscess, and with a manner both apologetic and authoritative, the doctor referred her promptly to a surgeon to drain what he hoped would be the last outpost of this grim and mysterious foe. His hopes were premature or ill-informed, for she soon developed a bowel complaint with loose, frequent motions and the passage of mucus. The hospital physicians, asked to assess this problem, investigated her story and internal tissues with zealous and impressive thoroughness, fearing that her relentless and severe constellation of complaints might be due to some concealed fault in her immune system. Perhaps to their disappointment, but to Alice's relief, they found nothing.

When she came to tell Dr D of her 'progress'(!) and her most recent hospital odyssey, the doctor listened with courtesy and concealed despondency, before embarking on a lame but well-intentioned ritual of 'performing' a physical examination: he could not hope to unravel this Gordian knot, but at least he could be seen to be conscientious in his efforts. With a consoling but clueless hand on her abdomen he said:

'Events have moved so quickly and unpredictably that I haven't had a chance to get to know anything about you, apart from your illness. But I've been wondering if there's anything in your life, worries or frustrations, that you think might have brought all this on.'

Alice's abdomen tensed as her breath stopped momentarily, and Dr D did not expect the succinctness of the reply:

'I think you've got something there, doctor. You know, I just can't settle into this second marriage…'

Realizing the pregnancy of Alice's confidence was likely to be both fragile and crucial to understanding her menacing afflictions, Dr D acknowledged the importance of her statement, but desisted from asking anything more explicit from her, instead inviting her for a longer appointment where she could, if she wished, unfold and reveal her personal world.

Until ten years previously Alice had regarded herself as happily married to Tom. Their sexual relationship had always seemed a celebration of this; vibrant, full-blooded, enlivening and tender. Tom's confession had come with horrific suddenness: with shame but conviction, he told of an affair he was having with Alice's cousin, a woman much loved and valued by Alice. In a conflagration of shock, hatred and grief, this apparently loving and companionable relationship became a bitter and empty ruin. Alice, shamed, resentful, and uncomprehending, became circumspect and prickly, directing what bruised love she felt safe to entrust, toward her two sons.

This turbulent and bleak period of her life was eased somewhat by a kindly and attentive, though somewhat phlegmatic, neighbour, Cyril. Cyril too, had recently suffered a painful and central loss through his wife's death from breast cancer. Now a childless widower in his middle years with no family around him, his loneliness was soothed and expunged by his growing acts of concern and protectiveness towards Alice, a widow of sorts, an injured soul-mate. The two became bonded by mutual commiseration. Her two sons, hungering for paternal presence and interest, accepted Cyril's good humoured and stable involvement with an almost incredulous joy and gratitude: they had expected to remain fatherless. Alice's siblings and, now elderly, parents, at first warily protective of Alice, grew steadily in their warmth, admiration and respect for this unassuming and devoted man. It all seemed like a miracle of restoration when Cyril proposed marriage, and Alice, to the joy of all those around her, accepted.

But Alice's secret and inner world rumbled, faintly at first, with a doubt she could not communicate. While her gratitude and affection for Cyril warmed her heart, her flesh remained dispassionate to his touch. Tom had been a vital and charismatic lover, who had rarely failed to arouse and satisfy her deep visceral hungers, and to her dismay Cyril's body had seemed waxy and lifeless; at this primal level she could find no love for him.

'At first I thought I could grow to love him in that way, that it would come if I was patient. He's been so good to me and the children – the boys adore him. And I kept thinking: "It's not much to do in return. I should be able to offer him the sexual love he wants". But I just haven't been able to. At first I'd pretend, though it always hurt, and I tried to hide it. Then it got worse; I felt repelled and sick and terribly guilty for marrying him when I didn't desire him. It's a terrible problem I have, doctor. I can't reject him or leave him now, not after what he's done for me, and what he's been through with his wife dying. I think he'd die of a broken heart…'

'And the terrible infection you developed was like a way of keeping him out, and killing yourself, without you having to tell him anything painful. It's as if your body expressed, and attempted to solve, your whole painful predicament,' Dr D pondered, realizing that such metaphor might seem bizarre or obscurely distasteful to many of his colleagues.

'Yes, that's just how I've felt. The doctors at the hospital seemed amazed at my condition, but all the way through it didn't really surprise me. Secretly I thought of it as a way out, and as a kind of punishment … It all made some kind of awful sense,' Alice replied with stoic and dark candour.

Dr D, gratified and deeply moved by his understanding of the deeply tragic nature of Alice's dilemma, found himself feeling disorientated and impotent with his wish to help further. Toward the end of their harrowingly intimate hour together, realizing that the severity and momentum of this woman's problem was quite beyond his usual scope of support and clarification, the doctor suggested that her problem should be shared further with a counsellor.

'No, doctor,' she said with firm conviction. 'I can't tell anyone else, and I know nobody can do anything to change my situation. But you've probably done more than you realize, because it's important that someone, just one person, knows my situation and what I'm going through. It may sound strange, but it will help me manage. Can you understand that?'

Dr D's nod was warm and sorrowful. He did not need to say more.

Alice returned a fortnight later and reported her bowel complaint quiescent. Mindful of Alice's words on the previous occasion he did not enquire about her life, but the mellow and tender tone of the interview indicated that an implicit and important rapport had been created between them: she would return and talk if she needed to.

Dr D's 'psychotherapy' with Alice was not in any way complex or 'clever', the doctor merely provided a safe and attentive place where there was trust, time and containment enough for her to unburden herself in a way that was compassionately accompanied. Dr D, in allowing her to 'pour out' her secret pain and difficulties, had been struck by the way her bowel had no longer needed to fulfil this function symbolically and somatically. Putting her conflicts into words, it seemed, had thus shifted the locus of expression from her body.

There are other ways we can understand the healing encounter of Alice and Dr D In providing a 'Safe Space[11] for Alice to share her most anguished and burdensome secrets, she could, if only in that particular setting, bring together the self that was normally presented to the world and the self that she alone knew. From Freud onwards psychoanalysis has concentrated on the integration of the Conscious and Unconscious Self as the major task of psychological growth and healing. But the example of Alice illustrates a challenge more common in medical practice and counselling: for the integration of the split between her outer, Public Self and her inner, Secret

Self, is in no way 'unconscious', and yet is cardinal to her difficulties.[12]

Dr D's skill here did not lie in subsuming her communications to his own specialist concepts and frame of reference,[2] but rather to create the kind of relationship and dialogue where Alice was 'encouraged' in entrusting and accepting herself. This could only happen if she felt she could trust, and be accepted by, Dr D; and the doctor could create this kind of 'holding environment'[13] only if he could manage a particular kind of unconditional listening and responsiveness.[14] This is more complex than it might seem for, as we have seen with Dr B in Case No 2., such qualities of outer listening to another emerge from the long gestation of listening to oneself. The empathy mustered by Dr D could not arise merely from curiosity and benevolent intentions; the resonance required demanded a deep and hard-earned inner sentience.

Alice's final communications to Dr D at the end of her long interview have an intriguing and instructive message in the endeavour of psychotherapy. In a culture and profession increasingly obsessed with questions of active intervention, terminology and technique, we are, perhaps apt to overlook the healing power of being known, with intimacy and volition, to another.[15] It is often unmitigated aloneness that makes us sick; inclusion and acceptance that heal. It is here that the heart of the Alienist is most tested.

$$\Omega$$

References

[1] Balint, M. *The doctor, his Patient, and the Illness.* London: Pitman, 1957.

[2] Zigmond, D. Three types of encounter in the healing arts: dialogue dialectice and didacticism. *Holistic Medicine,* 1987; 2: 69-81.

[3] Bennet, G. *The Wound and the Doctor.* London: Secker and Warburg, 1987.

[4] Zigmond, D. Physician heal thyself: the paradox of the wounded healer. *Br J of Holistic Med* 1984; **1.**

[5] Steiner. C Emotional literacy. *Transactional Analysis Journal* 1984: 14

[6] See for example,
Alexander, F. Fundamental concepts of psychosomatic research: psychogenesis, conversion, specificity. *Psychosom Med* 1943; **5:** 205.

[7] Perls, F. *Gestalt therapy verbatim.* Utah: Real People Press, 1969.

[8] Zigmond, D. A psychosomatic approach. *Practitioner,* April 1982.
Zigmond, D. the psychosomatic mosaic. *Practitioner,* April 1982.

[9] See, for example
Bathrop, RW. Depressed lymphocyte function after bereavement. *Lancet* 1977; **1**: 834-6.
Selye, H. *The stress of life* New York: McGraw-Hill, 1956.
Friedman, SB, Glasgow LA, Ader R. Psychosocial factors modifying host resistance to experimental infections. *Ann New York Acad Sci* 1969; 164: 381-93.

[10] Balint, M. The basic fault. London & New York: Tavistock, 1968.

[11] Fry, A. Safe space. London: Dent, 1987.

[12] Zigmond, D. The elements of psychotherapy. *Practitioner* September 1981.

[13] Winnicott, D. *The maturational process and the facilitating environment.* New York: International Universities Press, 1965.

[14] Rogers, Carl *On becoming a person* New York: Houghton Mifflin, 1961.

[15] Pennebaker, JW, Becall, SK. Confronting a traumatic event: toward an understanding of inhibition and disease. *Abnormal Psychology* 95 274-81, 1986; 85: 274-81.

Publ. in *Holistic Medicine,* vol. 4, 197-208 (1989

The Author

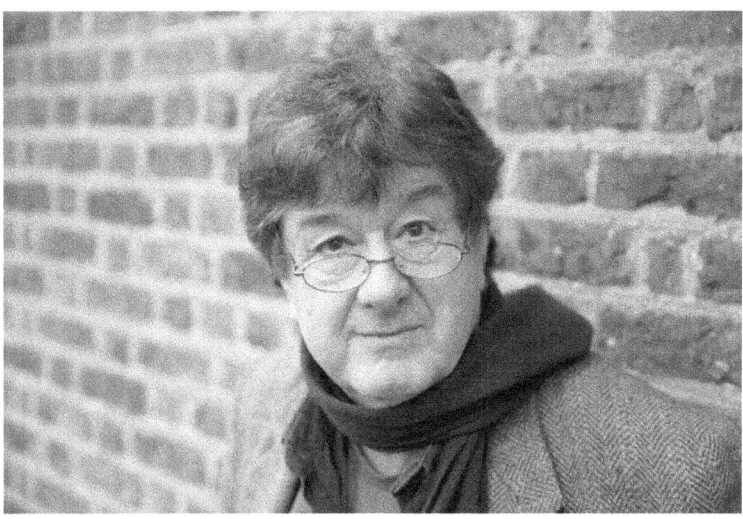

David Zigmond initially trained in Medicine in the 1960s. For several decades he has worked in the NHS as a small-practice GP, and as a large hospital psychiatrist and psychotherapist. Alongside these he has maintained a practice as a private psychotherapist. From these long tenures he has explored the nature and importance of relationships, imagination and personal meaning throughout healthcare. These have fuelled and guided his view and practice of holistic medicine. His long-spanned teaching and writing have been committed to develop and secure these values.

He helped launch the British Holistic Medical Association in the 1980s and has remained active in developing this approach. This anthology contains many of his contributions.

Other Books on Health by New Gnosis Publications

Wilberg, Peter *The Illness is the Cure - 2nd extended edition: an introduction to Life Medicine and Life Doctoring - a new existential approach to illness,* 2014

Wilberg, Peter *from Psychosomatics to Soma-Semiotics: Felt Sense and the Sensed Body in Medicine and Psychotherapy,* 2010

Wilberg, Peter *Being and Listening: Counselling, Psychoanalysis and the Ontology of Listening,*2013

Wilberg, Peter *Heidegger, Medicine and 'Scientific Method': The Unheeded Message of the Zollikon Seminars,* 2012

Wilberg, Peter *Meditation and Mental Health: an introduction to Awareness Based Cognitive Therapy,* 2010

Wilberg, Peter *The Therapist As Listener: Martin Heidegger And The Missing Dimension Of Counselling And Psychotherapy Training* 2008

Zigmond, David *If you want good personal healthcare – See a Vet Industrialised Humanity: Why and how should we care for one another?* (Complete collection, 716 p) 2015

Zigmond, David *From Family to Factory – Lost personal meaning in healthcare* (If you want good personal healthcare – See a Vet, Volume 2) 2015

Zigmond, David *Bureaucratyrannohypoxia - The struggle for personal meaning in healthcare* (If you want good personal healthcare – See a Vet, Volume 3) 2015

www.ingramcontent.com/pod-product-compliance
Lightning Source LLC
Chambersburg PA
CBHW051859170526
45168CB00001B/173